TEACHING INTERPERSONAL SKILLS

FORTHCOMING TITLES

Occupational Therapy for the Brain-Injured Adult
Jo Clark-Wilson and Gordon Muir Giles

Multiple Sclerosis
Approaches to management
Lorraine De Souza

Physiotherapy in Respiratory Care
A problem solving approach
Alexandra Hough

Community Occupational Therapy with Mentally Handicapped People
Debbie Isaac

Management in Occupational Therapy
Zielfa B. Maslin

Keyboard, Graphic and Handwriting Skills
Helping people with motor disabilities
Dorothy E. Penso

Speech and Language Problems in Children
Dilys A. Treharne

THERAPY IN PRACTICE SERIES

Edited by Jo Campling

This series of books is aimed at 'therapists' concerned with rehabilitation in a very broad sense. The intended audience particularly includes occupational therapists, physiotherapists and speech therapists, but many titles will also be of interest to nurses, psychologists, medical staff, social workers, teachers or volunteer workers. Some volumes will be interdisciplinary, others aimed at one particular profession. All titles will be comprehensive but concise, and practical but with due reference to relevant theory and evidence. They are not research monographs but focus on professional practice, and will be of value to both students and qualified personnel.

Teaching Interpersonal Skills

A handbook of experiential learning for health professionals

PHILIP BURNARD, PhD

University of Wales College of Medicine, Cardiff

 CHAPMAN & HALL

London · New York · Tokyo · Melbourne · Madras

UK	Chapman and Hall, 2–6 Boundary Row, London SE1 8HN
USA	Chapman and Hall, 29 West 35th Street, New York NY10001
JAPAN	Chapman and Hall Japan, Thomson Publishing Japan, Hirakawacho Nemoto Building, 7F, 1-7-11 Hirakawa-cho, Chiyoda-ku, Tokyo 102
AUSTRALIA	Chapman and Hall Australia, Thomas Nelson Australia, 102 Dodds Street, South Melbourne, Victoria 3205
INDIA	Chapman and Hall India, R. Seshadri, 32 Second Main Road, CIT East, Madras 600 035

First edition 1989
Reprinted 1991

© 1989 Philip Burnard

Typeset in 10/12 Times by Mayhew Typesetting, Bristol
Printed in Great Britain by
St Edmundsbury Press Ltd, Bury St Edmunds, Suffolk

ISBN 0-412-34590-0

British Library Cataloguing in Publication Data

Burnard, Philip
　　Teaching interpersonal skills: a handbook of
　　experiential learning for health professionals.
　　(Therapy in practice; 10)
　　I. Title
　　305.9'362
　　ISBN 0-412-34590-0

For Sally, Aaron and Rebecca

Contents

Preface

Many books on the topic of interpersonal skills and experiential learning begin with a grave warning that only those who have received lengthy training should use experiential learning methods to teach interpersonal skills. That's rather like saying only a fully trained artist should attempt to paint. This book takes a different point of view. It argues that most people, given a little time and commitment, have the personal experience to enable them to help others to improve their interpersonal skills. This book is aimed at anyone in the health professions who is concerned about enhancing interpersonal competence, either their own or other people's. It also tells you how to achieve this aim. The chapters that follow offer both theory and guidance in practice. The book contains many practical illustrations of 'how-to-do-it' and a longer, illustrative package that tries to convey the running of a typical interpersonal skills workshop.

The first chapter is the most academic of the book. It offers a fairly detailed analysis of the concept of experiential learning: the notion of learning through personal experience and the notion on which this book is based. The second chapter offers the reader some practical examples of the wide range of experiential learning methods available to her and notes on how to use them in interpersonal skills training. The third chapter discusses examples of interpersonal skills for use in the health professions and argues that a thorough grounding in counselling skills can enable the health professional to develop other interpersonal skills.

The next few chapters offer details of how to organize, set up and run interpersonal skills training workshops and groups, with examples from practice. The final chapter supplies a range of clearly laid out exercises for use in such workshops and groups. The book closes with a detailed bibliography of further and recommended reading. The reader should find it useful as a source of material for further study and practice.

The author learned to use the approaches described in this book by using them in training a variety of health care professionals in counselling, experiential learning, stress management, group facilitation, managing change, self-awareness and curriculum development over a period of more than ten years. In writing this volume, he hopes that a variety of health professionals, from nurses to social workers and from occupational therapists to GP's will find the approach easier than they thought and will enjoy the experience of experimenting with the exercises and activities contained in it.

Whilst the book is primarily written for tutors, trainers and lecturers in the health professions, it may also be useful to the clinical practitioner who wishes to develop expertise in helping patients and clients to enhance their interpersonal skills. In the fields of social work, health visiting and psychiatric nursing, for example, there are numerous occasions on which the development of conversational and social skills can help improve personal performance and self-awareness. The awareness of basic counselling and group skills can also do much to improve the quality of communication between people in families and organizations.

Throughout the book there are short sections called 'Activities for Improving Interpersonal Skills in the Health Professions'. These are brief exercises and tips that may help to enhance your own skills or make you think of activities that you can use in your workshops. These are intended to serve as ideas to make you think about your own interpersonal performance and how you can bring new ideas to your teaching and training groups. The book may be read through at a sitting, dipped into for ideas or referred back to when planning courses and workshops. I welcome any comments you may have on the book or on how I may improve it.

Like many other writers, I still have difficulties in solving the problem of how to write in non-sexist language. I considered using 'they' as both singular and plural but that seemed clumsy. Alternate chapters of 'he' and 'she' seemed equally awkward. I have settled for using 'she' to describe the facilitator of interpersonal learning groups. Please read 'he' when this is appropriate.

Philip Burnard
Caerphilly,
Mid Glamorgan,
Wales.

1

Experiential Learning

We all learn from experience. That is not to say that we learn everything from experience nor to suggest that we always learn from experience. A moments reflection will reveal how often that is not the case! I am constantly horrified by how often I do the same things and make the same mistakes, and haven't learned much in the process. On the other hand, I am equally surprised how often I have learned the really important things in my life, not from books nor from being told things by other people, but from having had something happen to me that I have found interesting or important. This is **experiential learning**.

In this first chapter, the concept of experiential learning is explored and applied to the learning of interpersonal skills for use in the health professions. It will become clear that the most effective interpersonal behaviour is that which we learn as we live. We cannot learn to be interpersonally competent by reading books on the subject (even this one), nor by listening to lectures on the topic. Whilst human experience is very varied and complicated, there are some ways of structuring it that can make personal experience useful for enhancing the ways in which we talk and behave with other people. Since caring human relationships form the basis of almost all of the caring professions, it would seem that harnessing personal experience may turn out to be a particularly useful endeavour.

The chapter begins with a discussion of some definitions of experiential learning and noting how the concept of experiential learning may be applied in health care settings. The chapter then goes on to define three types of knowledge and offers a revised definition of experiential learning in terms of this theory. A historical view of the topic is then offered and finally, the particular characteristics of experiential learning are identified and enumerated.

EXPERIENTIAL LEARNING DEFINED

Experiential learning is learning through doing. It is also more than that; it is learning through reflecting on the doing. In all aspects of our actions, we have at least two choices: to just act or to notice how we act. It is only through noticing what it is that we do that we can hope to learn about ourselves and our behaviour. To 'just act' is to act blindly, unawarely; this is what happens when we do not learn from experience. In a sense, it is as simple as that: if we are to learn from what we do, we must notice what we do and reflect on it. To notice what we do is to allow ourselves to evaluate action and to choose the next piece of behaviour. This is living in a more precise way. Obviously we cannot notice our behaviour and actions all the time, but in terms of the relationships we have with our clients, we owe it to them to notice our behaviour more frequently than we may be doing at present. To do this noticing is to engage in what Heron (1973) calls 'conscious use of the self': using behaviour and the self in a conscious, therapeutic manner. To make conscious use of the self during interpersonal relationships is to enhance the likeliness of our relationships being therapeutic.

Two examples from practice may help here. First, John Davies, a busy GP is having problems at home. As a result he unthinkingly looks unapproachable to his patients. He frowns a lot and has a tendency to be rather abrupt with them. His patients, therefore, find it more and more difficult to talk to him and tend to keep their conversations with him to a minimum. He continues to be unaware of the effect that he is having on them because he remains distracted by his own problems.

Sarah Elliot, on the other hand, is another GP, who is also having domestic and marital problems. She, however, makes a conscious effort to leave those problems behind her when she goes to work. She also pays attention to how she presents herself to her colleagues and her patients, both in the way she dresses for work and also with regard to her 'body language'. She has learned to notice, to reflect on her behaviour and to make conscious use of self. Thus her patients feel better from talking to her and find her approachable. This positive effect on her patients also makes *her* feel better and makes it a little easier for her to face the domestic problems which she picks up again when she returns home.

There is a second sense of the term experiential learning. We all learn through experience, whether directly, through taking action, through being involved in a situation or by observing others. In this sense every situation is an experiential learning situation. To describe experiential learning in such broad terms, however, would be rather fruitless: it would make the concept so huge as to render it unmanageable. To make things a little clearer, we may identify three aspects of experiential learning:

1. personal experience;
2. reflection on that experience;
3. the transformation of knowledge and meaning as a result of that reflection.

A fourth stage, in which we use what we have learned, may also be added to the first three and thus a continuous cycle of experience–reflection–transformation of knowledge and meaning – action (experience), is created (Fig. 1.1).

Fig. 1.1. An experiential learning cycle.

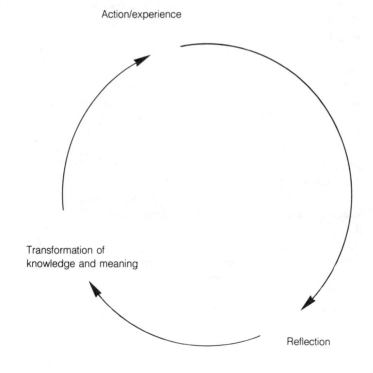

Action/experience

Transformation of
knowledge and meaning

Reflection

EXAMPLES OF EXPERIENTIAL LEARNING IN THE HEALTH CARE FIELD

All health professionals learn through reflecting on their practice. Experiential learning does not occur, as we have noted, when we do not reflect on our practice. The issue of reflection is a crucial one. In order to learn, we must first notice ourselves, or as the mystic, Ousepensky, (1988) put it, we must learn to remember ourselves. Ousepensky argues that for much of our lives we are only half conscious, or we are working on 'automatic pilot'. When we do this, we no longer register what is happening to us. Indeed, Ousepensky argues that if we do not remember ourselves and notice what is happening to us, we will not commit to memory the events that are taking place within and around us. We must learn instead to cultivate an increasing awareness of our senses and/or our changing thoughts, feelings and actions. Examples of how this **reflective ability** can help us to learn in the health professions are as follows:

Learning through talking to clients;
Working in the field;
Reflecting on past clinical experiences;
Comparing notes with other health care professionals;
Noticing personal thoughts, feelings and emotions;
Exploring feelings in small groups;
Attendance at experiential learning workshops;
Learning counselling and group therapy by working with clients;
Keeping journals and diaries;
Receiving positive and negative feedback from colleagues and peers;
Comparing past and present situations;

Using relaxation and meditational activities;
Consciously managing time;
Using problem-solving devices and strategies;
Entering into personal therapy/counselling;
Consciously trying new coping strategies;
Learning by 'sitting with Nellie': learning on the job;
Trial and error learning;
Learning by experimentation;
Reading about, then trying out, new ideas;
Consciously changing role;
Practising new interpersonal skills;
Learning group facilitation by running groups.

EXPERIENTIAL LEARNING AS THE DEVELOPMENT OF EXPERIENTIAL KNOWLEDGE

Another approach to appreciating the notion of experiential learning comes through discussion of types of knowledge. The three types of knowledge that go to make up an individual may be described as **propositional knowledge**, **practical knowledge** and **experiential knowledge** (Heron, 1981). Whilst each of these types is different, each is interrelated with the other. Thus, whilst propositional knowledge may be considered as qualitatively different to, say, practical knowledge, it is possible, and probably better, to use propositional knowledge in the application of practical knowledge.

Propositional knowledge

Propositional knowledge is that which is contained in theories or models. It may be described as 'textbook' knowledge and is synonymous with Ryle's (1949) concept of 'knowing that'; this is further developed in an educational context by Pring (1976). Thus a person may build up a considerable bank of facts, theories or ideas about a subject, person or thing, without necessarily having any direct experience of that subject, person or thing. A person may, for example, develop a considerable propositional knowledge about, say, midwifery, without ever necessarily having been anywhere near a woman who is having a baby! Presumably it would be more useful to combine that knowledge with some practical experience, but this does not necessarily have to be the case. This then is the domain of propositional knowledge. Obviously it is possible to have propositional knowledge about a great number of subject areas ranging from mathematics to literature, or from counselling to social work. Any information contained in books must necessarily be of the propositional sort.

Practical knowledge

Practical knowledge is knowledge that is developed through the acquisition of skills. Driving a car or giving an injection, therefore, demonstrates practical knowledge, though, equally, so does the use of counselling skills which involve the use of specific verbal and non-verbal behaviours and intentional use of counselling interventions as

5

described above. Practical knowledge is synonymous with Ryle's (1949) concept of 'knowing how', which was further developed in an educational context by Pring (1976). Usually more than mere 'knack', practical knowledge is the substance of a smooth performance of a practical or interpersonal skill. A considerable amount of health professional's time is taken up with the demonstration of practical knowledge – often, but not always, of the interpersonal sort.

Traditionally, most educational programmes in schools and colleges have concerned themselves primarily with both propositional and practical knowledge and particularly the former. Thus the 'propositional knowledge' aspect of a person is the aspect that is often held in highest regard. Practical knowledge, although respected, is usually seen as slightly less important than the propositional sort. In this way, the 'self' can become highly developed in one sense – the propositional knowledge aspect – at the expense of being skilled in a practical sense.

ACTIVITIES FOR IMPROVING INTERPERSONAL SKILLS IN THE HEALTH PROFESSIONS Number 1.

Awareness

Awareness is the simple process of noticing what is going on around you. Most of the time we are caught up with our own thoughts and feelings and fail to observe the world surrounding us. The conscious practice of 'staying awake' and noticing what we and others do, can help us to improve our interpersonal skills. We cannot change unless we choose to; we cannot change unless we notice what we do.

Experiential knowledge

The domain of experiential knowledge is knowledge gained through direct encounter with a subject, person or thing. It is the subjective and affective nature of that encounter that contributes to this sort of knowledge; the knowledge through relationship. Such knowledge is synonymous with Rogers' (1983) description of experiential learning and with Polanyi's concept of 'personal' knowledge and 'tacit' knowledge (Polanyi, 1958). If we reflect for a moment we may discover that most of the things that are really important to us belong in this domain. If for example we consider our personal relationships with other people, we discover that what we like or love about them cannot be reduced to a series of propositional statements and yet the feelings we have for them are vital and are part of what is most important in our lives. Most encounters with others contain the possible seeds of experiential knowledge. It is only when we are so detached from other people that we treat them as objects and no experiential learning can occur.

Not that all experiential knowledge is tied exclusively to relationships with other people. For example I had considerable propositional knowledge about America before I went there. When I went there, all that propositional knowledge was changed considerably. What I had known was changed by my direct experience of the country. I had developed experiential knowledge of the place. Experiential knowledge is not of the same type or order as propositional or practical knowledge. It is, nevertheless, important knowledge, in that it effects everything else we think about or do.

Experiential knowledge is necessarily personal and idiosyncratic; indeed, as Rogers (1985) points out, it may be difficult to convey to another person in words. Words tend to be loaded with personal (often experiential) meanings and thus to understand each other we need to understand the nature of the way in which the people with whom we converse use words. It is arguable, however, that such experiential knowledge is sometimes conveyed to others through gesture, eye contact, tone of voice, inflection and all the other non-verbal and paralinguistic aspects of communication (Argyle, 1975). Indeed, it may be experiential knowledge that is passed on when two people (for example a health visitor and her client) become very involved with each other in a conversation, a learning encounter or counselling.

As a development of the above discussion of three types of knowledge, it is possible to define experiential learning as any learning activity which enhances the development of experiential knowledge. Experiential learning, then is personal learning: learning that makes a difference to our self concept. As all interpersonal relationships with others, both within and without the health care professions involve an investment of self, it seems reasonable to argue that any learning methods that involve the self and that involve personal knowledge are likely to enhance personal effectiveness. We cannot, after all, learn interpersonal skills by rote, nor merely by mechanically learning a series of behaviours. We need to spend time reflecting on ourselves and on receiving feedback on our performance from other people. All of the experiential learning methods described in the next chapter involve these things.

THE HISTORICAL DEVELOPMENT OF THE CONCEPT OF EXPERIENTIAL LEARNING

Clearly, people have always learned from experience. However, the idea of experiential learning as an educational concept is a relatively recent one. It will be useful to review some of the historical roots of the concept in order to make sense of some of the experiential learning methods that follow in the next chapter.

Drawing on the work of American pragmatic philosopher, John Dewey (1916, 1938), Keeton *et al.* (1976) describe experiential learning as including learning through the process of living and include work experience, skills developed through hobbies and interests, and non-formal educational activities. This approach to definition is reflected in the FEU project report *Curriculum Opportunity* which asserts that, for the purposes of that report, experiential

Fig. 1.2 Experiential learning cycle (After Pfeiffer and Goodstein, 1982).

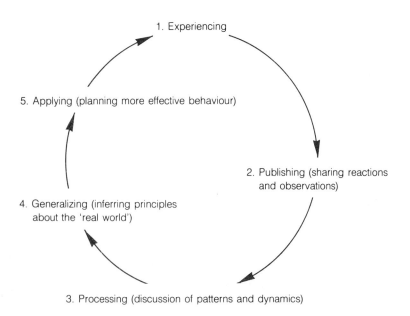

1. Experiencing

5. Applying (planning more effective behaviour)

2. Publishing (sharing reactions and observations)

4. Generalizing (inferring principles about the 'real world')

3. Processing (discussion of patterns and dynamics)

Fig. 1.3 Experiential learning cycle (After Kolb, 1984).

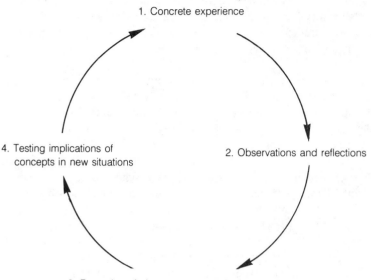

1. Concrete experience

4. Testing implications of concepts in new situations

2. Observations and reflections

3. Formation of abstract concepts and generalizations

learning referred to the knowledge and skills acquired through life and work experience and study (FEU, 1983).

Pfeiffer and Goodstein (1982) offer a different approach to the concept by describing an 'experiential learning cycle' which spells out the possible process of experiential learning (Fig. 1.2). This cycle not only suggests the format for organizing experiential learning but also makes tacit reference to the way in which people learn through experience.

Kolb (1984) was more explicit about this learning process in his 'experiential learning model' (Fig. 1.3). In this model, concrete experience is the starting point for a reflective process that echoes Paulo Freire's (1972) concept of 'praxis'. Praxis, for Freire, is the combination of reflection–and–action–on–the–world: a transforming process that is one of man's distinguishing features and one that enables him to change his view of the world and ultimately to change the world itself.

Malcolm Knowles, the American adult educator, took a different approach to the definition of experiential learning (Knowles, 1980). He described the activities that took place within the concept and thus listed the following, which he called 'participatory experiential techniques':

Group discussion, cases, critical incidents, simulations, role-play, skills practice exercises, field projects, action projects, laboratory methods, consultative supervision (coaching), demonstrations, seminars, work conferences, counselling, group therapy and community development.

His list seems so all-inclusive that he seems to have been saying that experiential learning techniques were any techniques other than the lecture method or private, individual study and that experiential learning was synonymous with participant and discovery learning. Boydel (1976) took just such a position when he asserted that:

Experiential learning in general terms is synonymous with meaningful discovery learning. This is learning which involves the learner sorting things out for himself by restructuring his perceptions of what is happening.

To summarize the position adopted by those writers who devised their definitions of experiential learning from the work of Dewey, would involve noting first the accent on some sort of cycle of events starting with concrete experience. It is worth noting that Kolb's and Pfeiffer and Goodstein's cycles were, in fact, anticipated by Dewey himself:

Thinking includes all of these steps, the sense of a problem, the observation of conditions, the formation and rational elaboration of a suggested conclusion and the active experimental testing. (Dewey, 1916)

The notion of learning from experience being a cycle involving action and reflection was a theme frequently echoed amongst modern writers (see, for example, Kelly, 1970; Hampden-Turner, 1966). Kolb's notion of transformation of experience and meaning can also be traced back to Dewey. He wrote that:

In a certain sense every experience should do something to prepare a person for later experiences of a deeper and more expansive quality. That is the very meaning of growth, continuity, reconstruction of experience. (Dewey, 1938)

This, then, was the influence on experiential learning from the Dewey perspective. The accent throughout, was on the primacy of

---

ACTIVITIES FOR IMPROVING INTERPERSONAL SKILLS IN THE HEALTH PROFESSIONS Number 2.

Self description

Try writing out a description of yourself in the third person. That is to say, start the description as follows . . . 'John Smith is an interesting person who . . .'. The process of doing this can add insight into how we perceive ourselves and how we think others perceive us. This activity can also be used as a group exercise. Each person writes out their own self-description and then shares it with the rest of the group. Each person may also ask for feedback on their particular description.

---

personal experience and on reflection as the tool for changing knowledge and meaning.

The other main influence on the development of experiential learning was the school of psychology known as 'humanistic psychology'. Humanistic psychology developed in the 1940s, '50s and '60s as a reaction to the 'mechanism' of behavioural psychology and the determinism of psychodynamic psychology. It argued that persons were free to choose their own lives and thus were 'authors' of their own existence. This philosophical perspective drew heavily on the existentialism of Sartre (1956), Heidegger (1927) and others. Humanistic psychology's main leaders, particularly in the 1960s (which offered exactly the right climate in which humanistic psychology could flourish) were Carl Rogers (1967) and Abraham Maslow (1972), who is said to have named humanistic psychology (Grossman, 1985). Rogers is particularly well known for his client-centred counselling and for his student-centred learning methods. Many of the experiential learning methods described below developed out of the school of humanistic psychology, which, rather like Deweyan educational practices, emphasized the uniqueness of human experience and human interpretation of the world. It should be noted, in passing, that Rogers had been considerably influenced by Dewey as he had been taught at university by a student of Dewey's, William Kilpatrick (Kirschenbaum, 1979). In this way we begin to develop a sense of experiential learning's heritage: American, (although drawing, also, from European philosophical traditions), with a heavy emphasis on personal experience and personal development.

THE PARTICULAR CHARACTERISTICS OF EXPERIENTIAL LEARNING

Moving on from the above discussion of experiential learning, the theory of knowledge and the historical perspectives, it is possible to draw out those characteristics that go to make up the approach to learning known as the **experiential approach**. These characteristics are offered as a further means of clarification and as the beginning of practical guidelines about how to use the approach in practice. In the next chapter, specific experiential learning methods will be described in detail.

In experiential learning there is an accent on action

Both the Dewey and the humanistic approaches to experiential learning involve the learner in action. This is not to say that the learner is 'doing something' in a trivial sense but that she is engaged in an activity that should lead to learning. This is in opposition to traditional teaching/learning strategies which require that the learner remain passive in relation to an active teacher who is the dispenser of knowledge. Freire (1972) has called this traditional approach the 'banking' approach to education: knowledge is delivered to the learner in chunks and the learner later 'cashes out' this information in examinations. The experiential learning approach is closer to Freire's concept of 'problem posing' education. Here problems are encountered through discussion, argument and action. The learner is no longer passive but in dialogical relationship with an equally active teacher.

There is a second, less important sense of action too. In experiential learning the learner is often physically moving to take part in structured activities, role play, psychodrama and so on, as opposed to more traditional learning situations in which the learner is sitting behind a desk or table.

Learners are encouraged to reflect on their experience

Most writers acknowledge that experience alone is not sufficient to ensure that learning takes place. Importance is placed on the integration of new experience with past experience through the process of **reflection** (Kolb, 1984; Kilty, 1983; Freire, 1972; Burnard, 1985).

Reflection may be an introspective act in which the learner alone integrates new experience with old. It may also be a group process whereby sense is made of an experience through group discussion. If reflection as a group activity is to be successful, the group leader is required to act as a group facilitator and may require special skills and knowledge. These skills and types of knowledge are discussed in later chapters of this book. It is suggested that the skills associated with group facilitation are different from the skills associated with the usual processes of teaching in that the group facilitator takes a non-directive or non-authoritarian stance in relation to the learners. In a reflective group, the leader as facilitator is not ascribing meanings to experience nor offering explanations but allowing learners to do these things for themselves.

A Phenomenological approach is adopted by the facilitator

Phenomenology may be defined as the description of objects or situations without their being ascribed values, meanings or interpretations. Phenomenology as a philosophy was developed by Husserl (1931) and underpins the philosophical writings of the existentialists (Sartre, 1956; Macquarrie, 1973).

The facilitator who uses a phenomenological approach restricts himself to the use of description as a means of summarizing what a learner has said and enables that learner to invest their own learning with meaning. The 'valuing' process is left to the learner. It is the learner who ascribes meaning to what is going on in the learning environment and the facilitator's meanings are not automatically foisted on the student. Reflecting this phenomenological approach, which eschews interpretation of experience by another person, Carl Rogers (1983) prefers to use the term 'facilitator of learning' rather than the more traditional terms 'teacher' or 'leader'. In using such a descriptor he hoped to remove the connotation of the teacher as expert or authority in the interpretation of experience. In the literature on experiential learning, the term facilitator is often used in preference to the terms teacher, lecturer, tutor or leader.

There is an accent on subjective human experience

Alfred North Whitehead (1932) discussed the problem of 'dead knowledge' and asserted that knowledge kept no better than fish!

The experiential approach to learning stresses the evolving, dynamic nature of knowledge. Rather than evoking R.S. Peter's (1972) notion of education as initiation into particular ways of knowing, it stresses the importance of the learner understanding and creating a view of the world in that learner's own terms. Postman and Weingartner (1969) noted that traditional education assumes a linear model of knowledge in which there is absolute truth and a single fixed reality. Citing anthropological evidence that our language tends to limit our view of reality (Worf, 1956) and that the means by which subject matter is communicated fundamentally alters the content of that communication, Postman and Weingartner challenge the linear view of education, claiming that learners need to develop the ability to ask critical questions about any so-called 'facts' that are presented to them. They quote Ernest Hemingway in suggesting (rather irreverently) that all learners should be encouraged to develop 'shockproof crap-detectors'!

Experiential learning allows for different means of communicating concepts, accounts for 'multiple realities' and invites critical reflection. In this respect, it differs considerably from the traditional model of education and training.

Human experience is valued as a source of learning

The accent in experiential learning, through its variety of learning methods and through its name, is on experience. Learners, as has been noted, are encouraged to reflect on past experiences to plan for future events. In formulating this concept of andragogy (the theory and practice of the education of adults), Malcolm Knowles (1978, 1980) stresses the value of experience in the sphere of adult learning. He maintains that as an individual matures so she accumulates an expanding reservoir of experience that causes her to become a rich source for learning. Knowles argues that the resource should be tapped in the educational process because, as Knowles puts it 'To an adult, his experience is *who he is*' (Knowles, 1978). Thus, for Knowles, there is an important ontological issue: an adult's experience is not something exterior and tacked on but is part of the person's self-concept. Experiential learning then is an attempt to make use of human experience as part of the learning process. It may be noted that the humanistic approach to experiential learning pays particular attention to the emotional aspect of the individual's experience (Heron, 1981).

Finally, whilst discussing the characteristics of experiential learning, it may be noted that what is under consideration is:

1. a set of teaching/learning methods, and
2. an attitude towards learning.

In the next chapter we will consider the range of experiential learning methods. The experiential learning approach as an attitude commends a model of education which stresses autonomous judgement, freedom of thought and the value of subjective human experience – values that may be supported by anyone working in the health professions.

2

Experiential learning methods for interpersonal skills training

A wide variety of learning methods have evolved, often out of the humanistic approach to the field, that have come to be known as **experiential learning methods**. All of these methods focus on the student or learner being offered an experience, followed by the reflection and the making sense of that experience, which was described in Chapter 1. In this chapter some of those methods are examined critically, and practical suggestions are offered for their use in interpersonal skills training. The methods differ from more traditional teaching methods (which usually involve some sort of 'telling' on the part of the teacher). Experiential learning methods all honour principles of experiential learning discussed in the previous chapter.

EXPERIENTIAL LEARNING METHODS

Pairs exercises

Pairs exercises, such as the ones described in Chapter 8, are particularly useful for learning and practising interpersonal skills such as counselling skills. The usual format for the pairs exercise is that each person nominates themselves 'a' or 'b'. Then 'a' practises the particular skill (for example, using open-ended questions) in the supportive presence of 'b'. After a period in these roles, the two people swap round and 'b' practises the skill in the supportive presence of 'a'. It is important that the exercise is *not* seen as a form of conversation but as a highly structured learning exercise. After each of the individuals has had a turn in the 'driving seat', the pair may spend time freely evaluating and appraising the exercise. Alternatively, the pair may rejoin a larger group to discuss the exercise with other people.

An alternative use of the pairs format is for the pair in question to take a theme and for one person to discuss that theme whilst the other person listens. After a prescribed time, the pair switch roles and the listener becomes the talker and vice versa. After an equal amount of time in this second phase of the activity, the pair may link up with another pair and discuss the issue in a foursome. Alternatively, they may be invited back into a larger group to discuss the issues in amongst all of their colleagues. Suitable themes and questions, related to health care and interpersonal skills development, include the following:

What do I need to do to enhance my interpersonal skills?
In what respects am I interpersonally skilled?
What do I need to do to improve my counselling skills?
What am I like as a teacher?
What are my personal strengths/weaknesses?
How well do I conduct interviews?
How do my colleagues see me?
How do my family see me?
What are the best and worst things about my relationships with my clients?
What are my strengths and weaknesses as a social/worker/ nurse/doctor etc.?

Examples of the use of the pairs method in health care training:

1. Physiotherapy: practising introducing self to new patients;
2. GPs: rehearsing terminating a consultation;
3 Speech therapy: practising offering and explaining new information to children.

Structured group activities

Structured group exercises allow for the experiential learning cycle to be worked through by a learning group. There are a number of publications (including this one) which describe a variety of group activities for enhancing interpersonal, social and counselling skills (Murgatroyd, 1986; Burnard, 1985). The idea of these activities is that the group undertakes an experience after which they discuss their thoughts and feelings about the experience and apply the new learning to the real or clinical situation. The advantages of this

17

approach include the sharing of a common experience, the generation of a wide range of possible solutions to practical problems and the realisation of both the personal and the common nature of group experience. Much can be learnt, experientially, about how to run and be members of groups by taking part in structured group activities. Many of the best structured group activities are those that the facilitator or the group devise themselves.

There are some important guidelines that may help in the smooth running of the structured group activities which may be identified as follows:

1. Full and clear instructions must be given to the group, and questions must be asked by the facilitator to establish that everyone in the group is clear about what to do.
2. Participation should always be voluntary and participants given the chance to sit out as observers.
3. Plenty of time must be set aside after the exercise in order to process or discuss the activity. Rushed processing of activities is a sure sign of an inexperienced facilitator.
4. The facilitator should be just that and not rush to offer his or her own explanations or interpretations of what has just happened in the group.
5. A debriefing period should follow the exercise to allow time for the participants to re-enter their normal, everyday roles.
6. The facilitator should encourage the group members to link any new learning with 'real life' and with their jobs away from the group. Group members should also be encouraged to practise any new skills learned, as soon as possible.

Examples of the use of structured group exercises in health care training:

1. Nursing: developing self-awareness in psychiatric nursing;
2. Social work: learning counselling skills;
3. Probation officers: learning appropriate assertiveness.

Role-play

Role-play involves the setting up of an imagined and possible situation, acting out that situation and learning from the drama (Fig. 2.1). More specifically, the cycle indicates that after a role-play, a period

Fig. 2.1 The stages involved in role-play.

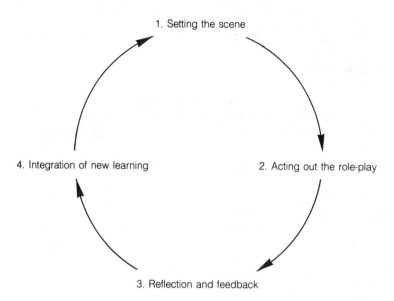

1. Setting the scene

4. Integration of new learning

2. Acting out the role-play

3. Reflection and feedback

of reflection is necessary, followed by feedback from other participants in order that new learning can be absorbed from the drama.

The first stage of a successful role-play, 'setting the scene', consists of inviting a number of participants to play out a scene, either from their own past or one they are likely to encounter in the future. Scenes replayed from the past are useful in that the role-play allows further reflection on those past situations. Anticipated scenes, on the other hand, allow for the rehearsal of new behaviour.

Once the 'players' have been selected, scenery and props of a simple sort should be used to create the invoked scene, for example tables and chairs suitably arranged.

Once scenery has been set and roles cast, the role-play can begin. The facilitator acts as 'director' and helps the actors to fully exploit their roles. Occasionally the facilitator may stop the role-play and allow a character to slow down her acting or take time out to consider how best to play the next part of the scene.

When the scene has been played out to the satisfaction of the players, the facilitator asks the players to reflect on their performances and those of their colleagues. An appropriate feedback order is as follows:

1. the principal actor self-reports on her performance;
2. the supporting actors offer the principal actor feedback on her performance;
3. the audience offers the principal actor feedback on her performance;
4. those three stages are repeated for all the other actors.

Following such feedback (which takes considerable time and should not be hurried), the role-play can be re-run and new learning, gained from the feedback, can be incorporated into the new performance.

Role-play is particularly useful for teaching and learning in the following domains of interpersonal skills training:

1. counselling skills training, (Nelson-Jones, 1981);
2. group facilitation training, (Heron, 1973);
3. assertiveness training, (Alberti and Emmons, 1982);
4. social skills rehearsal, (Ellis and Whittington, 1981).

Apart from the use of role play in the development of interpersonal skills, it may also be used as an aid to develop empathy; to rehearse initial practitioner/client meetings; to develop interview skills; to practise public speaking or the delivery of seminar papers and as a problem-solving activity. In this latter context, a problem situation is acted out with a variety of possible 'solutions'. The actors and the audience decide which solution feels best after they have completed the various role-plays.

What, then, are the limitations of role-play? The first limitation is that, by definition, role play is never real, it is always a simulation of a real situation. Unlike most other experiential activities, the participants are always asked to act either as though they were someone else or as though they were in a situation other than the present one. Some sense of the artificial will always be present.

Indeed, it can be argued that if this slight sense of unreality is not present, then the role-play is not working. If the situation cannot be distinguished from real life then the actors are no longer acting; they are reacting realistically in present time. This is fine as far as it goes, but it is not role-play.

A question mark must always hang over the issue of whether or not the behaviour participants exhibit in role-play bears any relation to the behaviour that they would exhibit in 'real life'. Role play takes place in a safe environment – very often in a college or a training department. The players are supported by their colleagues who watch knowing that what they see is play acting. In real life, neither the safe environment nor the supportive colleagues would necessarily be there. Who is to say that what someone does in role-play is in any way equivalent to what that person would do away from it? Just as we would not expect actors in a play to extend their roles into their lives away from the theatre, so we cannot guarantee any necessary continuity between performances in role-play and performance in the real health care setting. Acting is, after all, acting.

The second limitation is that role-play may appeal only to those who are extrovert enough to take part in it. It seems likely that those who observe the role-play gain considerably from looking on, through vicarious learning, but there is no substitute for taking part. Acting, however, does not appeal to everyone. Some participants may be unable to enter into a role or have no particular wish to do so. While such reservations must be honoured by the facilitator, they must call into question the validity of the method.

Another more complicated limitation may also arise here. The anxious-to-please participant or unassertive participant may agree to take part in order to please the facilitator. Alternatively, such a participant may feel compelled to take part because of group pressure. It is naive to think that all the facilitator has to do is tell the group that no one *has* to take part and that the decision by a participant not to take part will be fully honoured. Group dynamics and individual psychologies are more complex than that. The need to please the facilitator or other group members may override individual needs and wants.

Finally comes the question of transfer of learning. It has been acknowledged that role-play can never be real life. It is always an approximation, a symbolic representation. Can we assume, therefore, that the skills developed through role-play necessarily transfer over into the real health care setting? One may hope that they do but such hope can never amount to a guarantee. What we are asking is that skills learned in an artificial setting be used in a real setting. It may just be that the disjunction between the artificial and the real is too great.

It is important to differentiate between role-play and skills rehearsal. Role-play, as we have seen, involves inviting people to play out roles other than their own. Skills rehearsal, on the other hand, is where skills such as counselling and group facilitation are practised but with the person remaining as who she is at the present time. A typical example of skills rehearsal is the pairs exercise format described above. Thus a pairs exercise which develops listening

21

skills through one person consciously giving her attention to another, while the other talks, is skills rehearsal; it is not role-play. This important difference is sometimes blurred. The criticisms that may be levelled at role-play are not necessarily true of skills rehearsal. These then are some of the limitations of role-play. Having stated them it is important to acknowledge, also, that used wisely, role-play remains a useful method of activity involving participants in their own learning. If it is necessary to 'try out' new behaviours and new skills before working in the field (and it seems difficult to argue otherwise), role-play offers a valuable vehicle for such practice. What are offered now are some practical guidelines for running role-plays.

Role-play is rather different from structured group exercises in that in a role-play the participants are invited to enter different roles from their normal ones and to try out new behaviour. It is helpful if participants volunteer for particular roles. Definite stages in the role-play process may be identified as follows:

1. Explanation, by the facilitator, of the aims of the role-play. Sometimes this aim is negotiated within the group or identified as likely to be useful by a small number of group members.
2. Agreement about roles to be played out.
3. Outlining of possible scripts. This stage is optional; some groups prefer to ad lib the role-play.
4. The acting out of the role-play.
5. Evaluation of their performances by the main characters in the role-play.
6. Evaluation of the performances by any observers in the group (those members not directly taking part in the role-play).
7. Discussion and processing of the role-play with a full discussion of how everyone felt.
8. If required, a re-enactment of the role-play to allow for changes in performance. This is particularly useful in assertiveness groups and counselling skill groups where brand new skills are being rehearsed. The second performance can often allow performers to add to their skills by taking account of the discussion generated by the first role-play.

Examples of the use of role-play in health care training:

1. Social work: preparing to work with abused children;
2. GPs: anticipating counselling depressed patients;

3. Occupational therapy: practising planning rehabilitation with patients.

Psychodrama

A variant of role-play is psychodrama (Moreno, 1959, 1969, 1977). In psychodrama, a 'real life' situation that has been lived by one or more of the group members is re-enacted and then discussed by those actors and by the group. The above stages are worked through in psychodrama in much the same ways as they are in standard role-play. Slight variations in approach may be noted, however, and the following stages offer a more complete guide to the process of psychodrama:

1. The scene to be replayed is selected.
2. The main actor, who has described the scene to be re-enacted, chooses fellow actors from the group to play other parts.
3. The main actor briefs those actors about their roles and gives them a clear outline of what happened in the real situation.
4. The psychodrama scene is played out. The main actor may stop the action to suggest small changes in performance. The aim is to recreate, as completely as possible, the past scene.
5. The performance is then processed by the group of actors and ideas are offered by any onlookers.
6. After the discussion, the situation is replayed *as the main actor would have liked it to have occurred*. This is a vital part of psychodrama in that it allows a second chance at playing out a situation and an opportunity for trying out new skills in a 'real' situation. Again, psychodrama is particularly useful for encouraging the development of assertiveness and counselling skills. It may also be used for exploring group members personal life problems. In this context, however, it should be used with caution and preferably only by someone experienced in the medium. Both psychodrama and role-play can invoke considerable emotion in both players and observers.

Examples of the use of the psychodrama in health care training

1. Voluntary workers: helping in deciding when to refer on to other health professionals;
2. Nursing: reflecting on working with dying patients and bereaved relatives;

3. Physiotherapy: enhancing performance when working with severely injured young people.

ACTIVITIES FOR IMPROVING INTERPERSONAL SKILLS IN THE HEALTH PROFESSIONS Number 3.

Suspending judgement

Notice how an internal censor tends to divide up into right and wrong what other people say. Try suspending judgement on other people until you fully hear what they say. Even then, try to remain non-judgemental! This skill is one of the basic prerequisites of effective counselling.

Brainstorming

The process known as **brainstorming** has frequently been cited as an example of a student-centred or experiential learning method (Heron, 1973; Kilty, 1983; Brandes and Phillips, 1984).

The basic method of brainstorming may be described as follows: The learning group is encouraged to consider a particular topic and to call out words that they associate with it. These words are then collated on to either a black or white board or onto a series of flip-chart sheets. If the sheets are used they can be hung around the room to form a series of posters that serve as *aides-memoire*. During this initial process of 'calling out' of associations, the group is encouraged not to discount any association – often the more bizarre ones can lead to creative thinking (Koberg and Bagnall, 1981).

This process of encouraging associations can be a short one, taking, perhaps, up to 5 or 10 minutes, or it can evolve into a lengthy session of up to 40 minutes, as a means of investigating a topic in depth. The noting down of associations in this way can be an end in itself. The activity can lead into a discussion or a more formal lesson. In this sense brainstorming is used as a warm-up activity to encourage initial thought about a topic.

A further elaboration of the process so far described is for the facilitator or tutor to work through the lists of words, with the group, crossing out obviously inappropriate words. This is more difficult than it sounds! Often what seems inappropriate to one person is important to another.

24

Following this second process, the facilitator can then work through the lists again, with the group, in order to **prioritize** items. Prioritizing is the process of putting the items into some sort of rank order. This may mean that the items are sorted along a dimension of 'most appropriate' words to 'least appropriate' words. Out of this activity can arise the subject matter for a discussion or a more formal session. The prioritized list that emerges from this activity can serve as a programme for the next session.

Another method of prioritizing is to invite group members to examine the lists and to place a pre-determined number of ticks against items that interest them most. Again, this method can be used to organize the next part of the programme or to determine the subject matter for the rest of the day, week, or even workshop.

This, then, is the basic method of brainstorming with various slight additions to make its use more extensive. The approach described above may be used in various ways. First, as we have seen, it can be used as a method of determining the content of a course. It can be used at the beginning of a workshop or on the first day of a block of training. Used this way it ensures that the course is truly grounded in the needs and wants of the students. In this way too, it draws upon students' prior knowledge and experience and may therefore be described as an experiential learning method (Hanks, Belliston and Edwards, 1977).

Second, the basic method may be used as a problem-solving device (Open University, 1987; Koberg and Bagnall, 1981). Faced with a particular clinical or practical problem in a group discussion, the facilitator may use the brainstorming approach to identify a wide range of ways of solving the problem. Again this method calls upon the learner's prior experience and it can encourage the reinforcement of learning through practical application. It can also encourage assertive behaviour in that learners see their solutions written up in front of them as viable propositions.

Third, the basic method can be used as an evaluation device. At the end of a workshop or block the group is encouraged to identify their associations regarding what they have learned. These can be identified under headings such as 'knowledge' and 'skills'. Again the process of prioritizing through the use of participants ticks can be used to identify the degree of agreement on areas of learning. The outcome of this use of brainstorming can be that new material is identified for the next learning session.

If the method is used as an evaluative process, it is important that plenty of time is set aside for the activity. In this way all aspects of learning can be identified. If the process is rushed, only the very obvious and superficial aspects of learning will surface.

Used in this way, brainstorming becomes a joint evaluation/assessment process; evaluation in that it encourages a value to be placed on what has been learned so far and assessment in that it identifies new areas for programme planning. The process is also clearly student-centred. It encourages the learners to identify what they have learned without the tutor anticipating particular areas of learning. It is worth noting however, that Patton (1982) points out that evaluation and assessment carried out in this way needs to be a very structured activity if it is not to degenerate into a 'free for all'. The tutor using this approach to evaluation needs to consider their level of skills in group facilitation in order to ensure that the evaluation is both systematic and effective.

Another way of using brainstorming is to consider it as a method of exploring feelings – the affective domain. Much has been written recently about the need for health professionals to develop self-awareness (Bond, 1986; Burnard, 1985; Jenkins, 1987). Part of this self-awareness development comes through identifying how we feel about something. Thus brainstorming can become a self-awareness instrument. Two examples of its use in this way can be described.

First, it can be used as a spontaneous activity during a more formal learning session. Thus, during a session on caring for the dying person, the tutor can gently encourage the group to brainstorm their feelings about the topic. Out of such a session can arise areas of personal difficulty or interest and these issues can be used as topics for further discussion. Disclosure of feeling states can also enhance self-awareness (Jourard, 1964, 1971).

Second, it can be used more directly as an 'affective activity' in its own right. Thus, the tutor sets out to explore with the group their feelings about a particular topic. For example, a group of psychiatric nursing students considering the topic of depression may be asked to identify their own feelings when they have felt depressed. Again, by drawing upon the student's own past experience, used in this way brainstorming is an excellent example of an experiential learning method. This particular format is useful for exploring more 'personal' aspects of the curriculum: spirituality, sexuality, interpersonal relationships, value and belief systems and so forth.

Finally, two variants of the basic method of brainstorming may be considered. One, is the use of brainstorming as a small group activity (Newble and Cannon, 1987). Students are invited to form small groups of three to five members. In each group, a facilitator or chairperson is elected and that person serves as the one who writes down the associations on flip-chart sheets. After a period of about 15 minutes, the small groups re-form and a plenary session is held. In this session, each group pins up their sheets and all other participants are invited to view the displayed sheets. Out of this viewing period evolves a discussion of a more general sort. The advantage of this approach to brainstorming is that it allows almost everyone to take part. Students who are more reticent in a large group may feel more comfortable working in the small groups.

The second variant on the basic approach is that of 'individual' brainstorming. Here students are encouraged to sit quietly on their own and to write down all the associations that they make on a particular topic. When a given period of time has passed (usually between five and ten minutes) those students may be invited to form a plenary session. In this session two things may be done. One is to discuss the process of the activity, i.e. what it felt like to carry out the activity. Second is to invite students to share what they have written down. This, again, must be a voluntary activity. Some of the jottings may be of a personal nature and group members may or may not wish to share them with the whole group.

Used in this way, the process of brainstorming becomes akin to the process of free-association – the basic activity of psychoanalysis (Hall, 1954; Bullock and Stallybrass, 1977). Perhaps because of this, strong feelings may, again, be identified and it is recommended that tutors using this method develop skills in handling emotions. It should be emphasized, of course, that this form of brainstorming is only similar to one aspect of psychoanalysis. Clearly it is nothing to do with psychoanalysis itself, in that psychoanalysis is a structured and lengthy therapeutic process that involves interpretation, by a trained analyst, of the associations made by the client. It is not suggested that brainstorming should evolve into a form of do-it-yourself psychoanalysis!

Certain principles emerge out of all the different sorts of brainstorming activities described here and out of the literature cited above. They may be enumerated as follows:

1. Keep it simple but keep it structured. Instructions need to be given clearly and be easily understood. The structure of the activity serves to keep that activity focused.
2. Keep to time. If the activity overruns it may appear loose and unstructured; if it underruns, it may appear rushed.
3. Ensure that all associations are written down exactly as they are

offered by the students. It is important that the tutor does not offer an 'interpretation' of students' offerings.
4. Allow everyone to have their say. It is important that domination by one student is kept to a minimum and that all feel free to talk.

Examples of the use of brainstorming in health care training
Brainstorming has wide application in almost all teaching and learning situations. It is particularly useful in identifying individual student groups' reactions to various situations, such as:

1. Working with the mentally handicapped;
2. Coping with bereavement;
3. Feelings about patients' or clients' sexuality;
4. Identifying career moves or prospects.

Six Category Intervention Analysis

Six Category Intervention Analysis (Heron, 1975, 1986), developed out of previous work by Blake and Mouton (1976), is a device for identifying possible types of effective interpersonal interventions between practitioners and clients of various sorts. It is also particularly useful as an interpersonal training tool.

The categories identified in Heron's category analysis are: prescriptive; informative; confronting; cathartic; catalytic; supportive. The main characteristics of these categories are outlined in Fig. 2.2. Heron further subdivides the categories under the headings **authoritative** categories and **facilitative** categories. Authoratitive interventions are those which enable the practitioner to maintain some degree of control over the relationship ('I tell you', interventions), and include the prescriptive, informative and confronting categories. Facilitative interventions are those that enable the locus of control to remain with the client ('you tell me', interventions), and include the cathartic, catalytic and supportive categories (see Fig. 2.3).

Heron claims that the category analysis offers an exhaustive range of therapeutic interventions. He further claims that the interpersonally skilled person is one who can move appropriately and freely between the various categories when using the category analysis as a means of guiding therapeutic action. Heron suggests that no category is more or less important than any other category. Paradoxically, however, he argues that catalytic interventions form a 'bedrock' type of intervention that may serve as the basis for

Fig. 2.2 Synopsis of the Six Category Intervention Analysis

Category	Nature of intervention
Prescriptive	To offer advice, make suggestions etc.
Informative	To give information, instruct, impart knowledge etc.
Confronting	To challenge restrictive or compulsive verbal or non-verbal behaviour.
Cathartic	To enable the release of tension and strong emotion through tears, angry sounds etc.
Catalytic	To be reflective, to 'draw out' through the use of questions, reflections etc.
Supportive	To offer support, be validating, confirming of the persons self-worth.

Fig. 2.3 Authoritative and facilitative categories

Authoritative categories	Facilitative categories
Prescriptive	Cathartic
Informative	Catalytic
Confronting	Supportive

effective communication and counselling. He also offers the view that because we live in a 'non-cathartic society' (Heron, 1977), where the overt expression of strong emotion is not highly valued, the cathartic category will tend to be less frequently and less skilfully used by many practitioners. Fielding and Llewelyn (1987) also note that there are different degrees of resistance to the overt expression of emotion influenced by culture within the UK. Heron goes on to make a case for the therapeutic value of cathartic release – a highly pertinent and contentious argument but one which is beyond the remit of this book. Suffice it to say that other commentators may not view cathartic release as being of such importance. George Kelly, for example, in acknowledging the need to 'look forward' in life rather than to look back at past traumas, says 'the only valid way to live one's life is to get on with it' (Kelly, 1969).

The category analysis is pitched at the level of intention. That is to say that it does not pick out a range of specific verbal behaviours but attempts to guide the user's intentions in making therapeutic interventions. Thus it is in no sense a mechanical behavioural training device but a means of enabling the user to discriminate between a range of varied therapeutic (and, by implication, non-therapeutic) interventions. The question remains, however, as to the degree to which trainers can have access to people's intentions and whether or not people can remember their intentions, after the event! The word 'intervention' is used here to describe any verbal or non-verbal statement or behaviour that the practitioner may use in the therapeutic relationship. The word 'category' is used here to denote a range of related interventions.

Heron's analysis offers a starting point for training and research into interpersonal skills. Like all theoretical frameworks, it remains open to revision in the light of experience and research. It is also important to note that Heron's category analysis is not a behavioural analysis in the sense that it breaks down interpersonal skills into microskills. Instead it aims at identifying people's intentions when engaging in interaction. This analysis of intentions must pose difficulties when attmepting to quantify people's views of what they are doing when they engage in human interaction. The whole issue of intentionality is a difficult one and some of the problems in this field are discussed elsewhere (Searle, 1983).

The category analysis can be used in the following ways:

1. As a means of identifying therapeutic interventions in counselling, teaching, group work and management.
2. As a method of appreciating the range of therapeutic intervention.
3. As a training tool. Interventions in each of the six categories can be rehearsed in interpersonal skills training as a means of developing competence.
4. As a research tool. The author has used the category analysis as a means of helping nurses to identify their strengths and weaknesses throughout the range of categories. In a recent piece of research which used the analysis as a self-rating scale (Burnard and Morrison, 1988), in a study of more than 80 trained nurses it was found that most of those nurses perceived themselves as being more skilled in being prescriptive, informative and supportive and least skilled in being catalytic, cathartic and confronting. The study was repeated with a larger group of student nurses and the same profile emerged (Burnard and Morrison, 1988). Heron (1975) anticipated that health care professionals would be more skilled in the prescriptive, informative and supportive categories and less skilled in being catalytic, cathartic or confronting.
5. As an evaluation tool for determining effectiveness across a wide

range of therapeutic interventions.

Examples of the use of Six Category Intervention Analysis in health care training

1. Social work and nursing: learning counselling skills;
2. Voluntary workers: learning telephone counselling skills;
3. Physiotherapy: working with patients' emotion release.

These are a range of experiential learning methods that have wide application in the field of interpersonal skills training in the health professions. In later chapters we will consider how best such methods may be used, how to set them up, how to plan their use in a curriculum and how to evaluate their effectiveness as instruments of learning. Before that, it will be helpful to consider the range of interpersonal skills that may be useful to all health professionals.

3

Identifying and learning interpersonal skills

The need for interpersonal skills in health professionals is clear and easily articulated; we need them in order to get on with others and to help them. As Martin Buber (1958) at length points out: we exist as selves-in-relation; we need other people as much as they need us. Not to be interpersonally skilled as a health care professional is to be ineffective as a health care professional. If you did not believe that interpersonal skills are important, it is doubtful that you would be reading this book.

The range of what constitutes interpersonal skills is vast. A short list of such skills would include at least the following: counselling; group membership skills; assertiveness; social skills; interviewing skills of various sorts; writing skills; using the telephone and group facilitation skills. Examples of how such skills are used in the health care setting are also numerous and a few would include the following:

1. Counselling skills: talking to the distressed or depressed client, discussing work issues with a colleague.
2. Assertiveness skills: coping with the 'difficult' client, working within a bureaucracy.
3. Social skills: dealing with the general public, introductions to clients, visiting clients in their own homes.
4. Facilitation skills: running groups for educational purposes, facilitating therapy groups.

All health care professionals need and use a variety of interpersonal skills in every aspect of their work. The difficult thing, however, is how to teach these skills to other people. Very often, they are learned through the process known as 'sitting with Nellie': the new health care professional is supposed to pick up various skills through observing older and more experienced colleagues at work. The second problem arises when those colleagues demonstrate that they do not have particular interpersonal skills! Arguably, again, this situation has arisen because those colleagues were also given no formal training and so the cycle of events is complete. This chapter sets out to explore how interpersonal skills may be taught to health care professionals.

Prior to any discussion about the skills themselves comes an appreciation of certain personal qualities that are a necessary prerequisite of effective interpersonal relationship. A basic cluster of such necessary qualities may be identified as warmth and genuineness, empathy and unconditional positive regard (Rogers, 1967). These personal qualities cannot accurately be described as 'skills' but they are necessary if we are to use interpersonal skills effectively and caringly. They form the basis and the bedrock of all effective human relationships.

ACTIVITIES FOR IMPROVING INTERPERSONAL SKILLS IN THE HEALTH PROFESSIONS Number 4.

Naive phenomenology

This refers to the notion of suspending the development of theories. As we go through life, especially if we have had a psychological, sociological or political training, we tend to theorize about what we or other people are doing. Try, for a period, merely to observe other people and resist the temptation to slot what they do into a particular theory. This activity can help to sharpen up observational skills and help to improve descriptive ability. It does not, of course, have any predicative power!

PERSONAL QUALITIES FOR INTERPERSONAL EFFECTIVENESS

Warmth and genuineness

Warmth in the health care relationship refers to an ability to be approachable and open to the client. Schulman (1982) argues that the following characteristics are involved in demonstrating the concept of warmth: equal worth; absence of blame; nondefensiveness; closeness. Warmth is as much a frame of mind as a skill and perhaps one developed through being honest with yourself and being prepared to be open with others. It also involves treating the other person as an equal human being. Martin Buber (1958) discusses the difference between the 'I–it' relationship and the 'I–thou' (or 'I–you') relationship. In the I–it relationship, one person treats the other as an object, as a thing. In the I–thou relationship, there occurs a meeting of persons, transcending any differences there may be in terms of status, background, lifestyle, belief or value systems. In the I–thou relationship there is a sense of sharing and of mutuality, a sense that can be contagious and is of particular value in the health care relationship. Meyeroff describes this well in his classic book on caring:

> In a meaningful friendship, caring is mutual, each cares for the other; caring becomes contagious. My caring for the other helps activate his caring for me; and similarly his caring for me helps activate my caring for him, it 'strengthens' me to care for him. (Meyeroff, 1972).

What is not clear is the degree to which a health care relationship can be a mutual relationship. Rogers (1967) argues that the health care relationship can be a mutual relationship but Buber acknowledges that because it is always the client who seeks out the health care professional and comes to that health care professional with problems, the relationship is, necessarily, unequal and lacking in mutuality. For Buber, the professional relationship starts and progresses from an unequal footing:

> He comes for help to you. You don't come for help to him. And not only this, but you are *able*, more or less to help him. He can do different things to you, but not help you . . . . You are, of course, a very important person for him. But not a person whom he wants to see and to know and is equal to. He is floundering around, he comes to you. He is, may I say, entangled in your life, in your thoughts, in your being, your communication, and so on. But he is not interested in you as you. It cannot be. (Buber, 1966)

Thus warmth must be offered by the health care professional but the feeling may not necessarily be reciprocated by the client. There is, as well, another problem with the notion of warmth. We all perceive personal qualities in different sorts of ways. One person's warmth is another person's sickliness or sentimentality. We cannot guarantee how our 'warmth' will be perceived by the other person. In a more general way, however, 'warmth' may be compared to 'coldness'. It is clear that the 'cold' person would not be the ideal person to undertake helping another person in a health care setting! It is salutary, however, to reflect on the degree to which there are 'cold' people working in the health care arena and to question why this may be so. It is possible that interpersonal skills training may help this situation for it may be that some 'cold' people are unaware of their coldness.

To a degree, however, our relationships with others tend to be self-monitoring. To a degree we anticipate, as we go on with a relationship, the effect we are having on others and modify our presentation of self accordingly. Thus we soon get to know if our 'warmth' is too much for the client or is being perceived by him in a negative way. This ability to constantly monitor ourselves and our relationships is an important part of the process of developing interpersonal and counselling skills.

Genuineness, is also another important aspect of the relationship. In one sense, the issue is black and white: we either genuinely care for the person in front of us or we do not. We cannot easily fake professional interest; we must *be* interested. Some people, however, will interest us more than others. Often, those clients who remind us of our own problems or our own personalities will interest us most of all. This is not so important as our having a genuine interest in the fact that the relationship is happening at all.

On the surface of it, there may appear to be a conflict between the concept of genuineness and the self-monitoring alluded to above. Self-monitoring may be thought of as 'artificial' or contrived and therefore not genuine. The 'genuineness' discussed here, relates to the health care professional's interest in the human relationship that is developing between the two people. Any ways in which that relationship can be enhanced must serve a valuable purpose. It is quite possible to be 'genuine' and yet aware of what is happening; genuine and yet committed to increasing interpersonal competence.

A summing up of the notion of genuineness in the context of counselling and helping the health care professional was provided by Egan when he identified the following aspects of it:

You are genuine in your relationship with your clients when you:

1. do not overemphasize your professional role and avoid stereotyped role behaviours;

2. are spontaneous but not uncontrolled or haphazard in your relationships;
3. remain open and non-defensive even when you feel threatened;
4. are consistent and avoid discrepancies – between your values and your behaviour, and between your thoughts and your words in interactions with clients – while remaining respectful and reasonably tactful;
5. are willing to share yourself and your experience with clients if it seems helpful. (Egan, 1986)

Learning warmth and genuineness

Can a person learn to be warm and genuine? It is arguable that we have learned all our personal qualities so why should we imagine that a person is somehow 'naturally' warm and genuine or not as the case may be? Clearly these qualities cannot be learned in the same way as skills. They can, however, be developed through the person's awareness of them as qualities at all and through that person striving to pay attention to the other person, to forgo artifice and the adoption of a 'professional veneer'. If we are to truly help others, we cannot do so if we are trying to maintain a particular posture or trying too hard to be professional. We must, instead, come to the client as we are. We must learn to be ourselves.

Empathic understanding

Empathy is a relatively new term, apparently coined by Titchner in 1909 to translate the German term 'Einfuhlung' (Bateson and Coke, 1981). The term is usually used to convey the idea of the ability to enter the perceptual world of the other person; to see the world as they see it. It also suggests an ability to convey this perception to the other person. Kalisch (1971) defines empathy as 'the ability to perceive accurately the feelings of another person and to communicate this understanding to him'. Mayeroff describes empathic understanding from the point of view of caring for another person:

To care for another person I must be able to understand him and his world as if I were inside it. I must be able to see, as it were, with his eyes what his world is like to him and how he sees himself. Instead of merely looking at him in a detached way from outside, as if he were a specimen I must be able to be *with* him in his world, 'going' into his world in order to sense from 'inside' what life is like for him, what he is striving to be, and what he requires to grow. (Mayeroff, 1972)

Empathy is different from sympathy. Sympathy suggests 'feeling sorry' for the other person or, perhaps, identifying with how they feel. If a person sympathizes they imagine themselves as being in the other person's position. With empathy the person tries to imagine how it is to be the other person. Feeling sorry for that person does not really come into it.

The process of developing empathy involves something of an act of faith. When we emphathize with another person, we cannot know what the outcome of that empathizing will be. If we pre-empt the outcome of our empathizing, we are already not empathizing – we are thinking of solutions and of ways of influencing the client towards a particular goal that we have in mind. The process of empathizing involves entering into the perceptual world of the other person without necessarily knowing where that process will lead to. Martin Buber, mystic and writer on psychotherapy, summed this up well, this mixture of willingness to explore the world of the other without presupposing the outcome, when he wrote the following metaphor:

A man lost his way in a great forest. After a while another lost his way and chanced on the first. Without knowing what had happened to him, he asked the way out of the woods.

'I don't know', said the first. 'But I can point out the ways that lead further into the thicket, and after that let us try to find the way together'. (Buber, 1958)

Developing empathic understanding is the process of exploring the client's world with the client, neither judging nor necessarily offering advice. Perhaps it can be achieved best through the process of carefully attending and listening to the other person and, perhaps, by use of the skills known as **reflection** which is discussed in a later chapter of this book. It is also a 'way of being', a disposition towards the client, a willingness to explore the other person's problems and to allow the other person to express themselves fully. Again, as with all aspects of the 'client-centred' approach to caring, the empathic approach is underpinned by the idea that it is the client, in the end who will find their own way through and will find their own answers to their problems in living. To be empathic is to be a fellow traveller, a friend to the person as they undertake the search. Empathic understanding, then, invokes the notion of befriending.

There are, of course, limitations to the degree to which we can truly empathize. Because we all live in different 'worlds' based on our particular culture, education, physiology, belief systems and so forth, we all view that world slightly differently. Thus, to truly empathize with another person would involve actually becoming that other person. We can, however, strive to get as close to the perceptual world of the other by listening and attending and by suspending judgement. We can also learn to forget ourselves temporarily and give ourselves as completely as we can to the other person. There is an interesting paradox involved here. First, we need self-awareness to enable us to develop empathy. Then we need to forget ourselves in order to truly give our empathic attention to the other person.

ACTIVITIES FOR IMPROVING INTERPERSONAL SKILLS IN THE HEALTH PROFESSIONS Number 5.

Practising new behaviour

Try something new! Mostly we think of ourselves as only having a limited repertoire of behaviours because we have a certain, rather fixed, view of ourselves. In trying out a new way of acting and even try out exaggerated behaviour, we may learn something about our self-imposed limitations. The novelist, Kurt Vonnegut, once wrote: 'We are what we pretend to be . . .' (Vonnegut, 1969). Try pretending to be something different! This activity may be used in a group context and group participants may be encouraged to try out new behaviours for the duration of the workshop. Some people are surprised how easy it is to be different!

Learning empathy

Empathy can be developed through the use of experiential learning methods. Emphasizing, as they do, listening, the sharing of experience and a pluralistic view of the world, such exercises soon encourage group participants to pay attention to what someone else is saying and to resist the temptation always to compare my experience with your experience.

The simple listening exercises offered in the final chapter of this book are a good starting place for learning empathy. Beyond these exercises, too, is the need to develop consciously the ability to put ourselves into the frame of reference of the other person. As we have seen, to some degree this means forgetting ourselves, our belief and value systems and suspending judgement on what we hear. Our aim is not to criticize or to judge but to listen and understand what the other person is trying to convey.

Unconditional positive regard

Carl Rogers' phrase **unconditional positive regard** (Rogers, 1967), conveys a particularly important predisposition towards the client, by the health care professional. Rogers also called it 'prizing' or even just 'accepting'. It means that the client is viewed with dignity and valued as a worthwhile and positive human being. The 'unconditional' prefix refers to the idea that such regard is offered without any preconditions. Often in relationships some sort of reciprocity is demanded: I will like you (or love you) as long as you return that liking or loving. Rogers is asking that the feelings that the health care professional holds for the client should be undemanding and not requiring reciprocation. There is a suggestion of an inherent 'goodness' within the client, bound up in Rogers' notion of unconditional positive regard. This notion of persons as essentially good can be traced back at least to Rousseau's *Emile* and is philosophically problematic. Arguably, notions such as 'goodness' and 'badness' are social constructions and to argue that a person is born good or bad is fraught. However, as a practical starting point in the health care relationship, it seems to be a good idea that we assume an inherent, positive and life-asserting characteristic in the client. It seems difficult to argue otherwise. It would be odd, for instance, to engage in the process of counselling with the view that the person was essentially bad, negative and unlikely to grow or develop. Thus, unconditional positive regard offers a baseline from which to start the health care relationship. In order to further grasp this concept, it will be useful to refer directly to Rogers' definition of the notion as it relates to the counselling and the health care setting:

> I hypothesize that growth and change are more likely to occur the more that the counsellor is experiencing a warm, positive, acceptant attitude towards what is the client. It means that he prizes his client, as a person, with the same quality of feeling that a parent feels for his child, prizing him as a person regardless of his particular behaviour at the moment. It means

that he cares for his client in a non-possessive way, as a person with potentialities. It involves an open willingness for the client to show whatever feelings are real in him at the moment – hostility or tenderness, rebellion or submissiveness, assurance or self-depreciation. It means a kind of love for the client as he is, providing we understand the word love as equivalent to the theologian's term agape, and not in its usual romantic and possessive meanings. What I am describing is a feeling which is not paternalistic, nor sentimental, nor superficially social and agreeable. It respects the other person as a separate individual and does not possess him. It is a kind of liking which has strength, and which is not demanding. We have termed it positive regard. (Rogers and Stevens, 1967).

Unconditional positive regard, then, involves a deep and positive feeling for the other person, perhaps equivalent, in the health professions, to what Alistair Campbell has called 'moderated love' (Campbell, 1984). He talks of 'lovers and professors', suggesting that certain professionals profess to love thus claiming both the ability to be professional and to express altruistic love or disinterested love for others. It is interesting that Campbell seems to be suggesting that a health care professional can 'professionally care' or even 'professionally love' her client. The suggestion is also that the health professional has a positive and warm confidence in her own skills and abilities in the health care relationship. Halmos summed this up when he wrote:

'You are worthwhile!' and 'I am not put off by your illness!' This moral stance of not admitting defeat is possible for those who have faith or a kind of stubborn confidence in the rightness of what they are doing. (Halmos, 1965)

The health care relationship, for Halmos, is something of an act of faith. There can be no guarantee that the counselling offered will be effective but the health care professional enters the relationship with the belief that it will be. It is this positive outlook in the health care professional and this positive belief in the ability of the client to change for the better that is summarized in Rogers' notion of unconditional positive regard. Such an outlook is also supported by Egan who, in his 'portrait of a helper' says:

They respect their clients and express this respect by being available to them, working with them, not judging them, trusting the constructive forces found in them, and ultimately placing the expectation on them that they will do whatever is necessary to handle their problems in living more effectively. (Egan, 1986)

Learning unconditional positive regard

Learning not to judge others often comes through accepting ourselves. We judge others more harshly when we have not resolved various personal problems. We judge even more readily when we do not know what our personal problems are. It is suggested, again, that the route to learning unconditional positive regard may begin with the development of self-awareness. Whilst we cannot hope to totally sort ourselves out, as health professionals helping other people with their problems, it seems reasonable that we begin by at least becoming aware of some of our own.

INTERPERSONAL SKILLS IDENTIFIED

Now it is possible to identify certain core interpersonal skills and offer clear descriptions of the stages of training that may be offered in workshops aimed at developing those skills. The style of training is that based on the notion of experiential learning, discussed in the last chapter. The argument is that the only way to learn interpersonal skills is to engage in them. They can be lectured upon, discussed and generally dissected but they will not be effectively learned until the learner uses them. The recurrent theme throughout this chapter (and throughout this book) is how to offer people experiences that will help them to develop their own particular but effective style of interacting with others.

It will be noted that counselling skills are argued to be the bedrock type of interpersonal skill upon which all others are built. It is asserted that the health care professional who can learn to use a wide range of effective counselling skills is well on the way to being interpersonally competent. The fact that the person who is counselling has to deal with so many different aspects of the human condition suggests that the one who can counsel effectively is likely to be able to transfer those skills to a variety of other interpersonal situations.

COUNSELLING SKILLS

Counselling skills may be used in a variety of health care settings. They may be used to help the person who is suffering from a temporary emotional crisis or they may be helpful in caring for the person who has longer term problems in living. They may also be practical and useful as a set of interpersonal skills for everyday use in every client-practitioner situation. Counselling skills, after all, are not skills to be turned on and off according to the need but a 'way of being' with the client to enable them to communicate their thoughts and feelings more effectively. Counselling skills form the basis of all effective interpersonal relationships between the health care professional and the health care consumer, whatever the relationship between those two people. Further, the skills are essential ones for helping other colleagues. A short list of situations in which counselling skills are useful in all of the caring professions includes:

helping relatives to cope with bereavement;
working with children and adolescents;
helping families to work through problems;
discussing psychiatric difficulties and making decisions about when to 'refer on' to other health care professionals;
helping other colleagues;
teaching students to become counsellors.

Counselling skills may be divided into two sub groups: **listening** and **counselling interventions**. Listening involves not only giving full attention to the person being listened to but also that we be seen to be listening by the other person. Gerard Egan (1986) argues that in Western countries, the following behaviours are often associated with effective listening and may be practised in order to enhance listening ability.

1. Sit **squarely** in relation to the person being listened to. This can be taken both literally and metaphorically. If we are to truly listen to the other person we need to be able to see them and for them to see us, thus it is better that we sit facing them rather than beside them. We also need to 'face' them in the sense of not being put off by them nor daunted by them.
2. Maintain an **open** position. Crossed arms and legs can often suggest defensiveness. It is better, then, to sit comfortably and in a relaxed uncrossed position.

3. **Lean** slightly towards the person being listened to. Egan argues that this is usually perceived as a warm and interested gesture. On the other hand, it is important that the other person does not feel crowded by the listener.
4. Maintain reasonable **eye** contact. The eyes are a potent means of interpersonal communication (Heron, 1970). It is important that our gaze is 'available' for the other person.
5. **Relax** whilst listening. Listening does not have to involve rehearsing the next thing to be said. All that is needed is the listening itself. The relaxed listener helps the person being listened to, to relax.

Egan shows the acronym SOLER as a means of remembering these basic listening behaviours. The letters in the acronym are used to remember the key words in the cycle.

Listening forms the basis of all good counselling and, arguably, of all interpersonal relationships. If the health profession can learn to enhance her listening ability she will see an improvement in other interpersonal skills too. Not that listening can ever be a mechanical set of behaviours. It also requires that we are 'present' for the other person; that we are with them as fellow human beings and not purely as professionals doing a job.

The other sub group of counselling skills is that of counselling interventions: the things that the counsellor says in the counselling relationship. Before specific counselling interventions are discussed, consideration needs to be made of our disposition towards counselling or our 'philosophy' of counselling.

The term **client-centred**, first used by Carl Rogers (1951) refers to the notion that it is the client himself who is best able to decide how to find the solutions to their problems in living. Client-centred in this sense may be contrasted with the idea of 'counsellor-centred' or 'professional-centred', both of which may suggest that someone other than the client is the 'expert'. Whilst this may be true when applied to certain concrete 'factual' problems (housing, surgery, legal problems and so forth), it is difficult to see how it can apply to personal life issues. In such cases, it is the client who identifies the problem and the client who, given time and space, can find their way through the problem to the solution.

Steve Murgatroyd (1986) described the client-centred way of caring as follows:

1. a person in need has come to you for help;

2. in order to be helpful they need to know that you have understood how they think and feel;
3. they also need to know that, whatever your own feelings about who or what they are or about what they have or have not done, you accept them as they are – you accept their right to decide their own lives for themselves;
4. in the light of this knowledge about your acceptance and understanding of them they will begin to open themselves to the possibility of change and development;
5. if they feel that their association with you is conditional upon them changing, they may feel pressurized and reject your help.

First, the client comes to you for help, not to anyone else. Also, it is not you who comes to the client for help. An obvious point but nevertheless an important one because it highlights the fact that the counsellor/client relationship can never truly be one of equals. The second point is the equally important one that the client needs to be truly understood. The need for empathy – the ability to enter the other person's frame of reference, their view of the world – is essential here. What we need to consider now are ways of helping the person to express themselves, to open themselves and thus to begin to change. There is an interesting paradox in Murgatroyd's last point, that if the client feels that their association with you is conditional upon them changing, they may reject your help. Thus we enter into the counselling relationship without even being insistent on the other person's changing.

In one sense, this is an impossible position. If we did not hope for change, we presumably would not enter into counselling in the first place! On another level, the point is a very important one. People change at their own rate and in their own time. The process cannot be rushed and we cannot will another person to change (Frankl, 1975). Nor can we expect them to change and become more the sort of person that we would like them to be. We must meet them on their own terms and observe change as they wish and will it to be (or not, as the case may be). This sort of counselling is very altruistic. It demands of us that we make no demands of others.

Client-centred counselling is a process rather than a particular set of skills. It evolves through the relationship that the counsellor has with the client and vice versa. In a sense, it is a period of growth for both parties for both learn from the other. It also involves the exercise of restraint. The counsellor must restrain herself from offering advice and from the temptation to 'put the client's life right for him'. The outcome of such counselling cannot be predicted nor can concrete goals be set (unless they are devised by the client, at their request). In essence, client-centred counselling involves an act of faith; a belief in the other person's ability to find solutions through the process of therapeutic conversation and through the act of being engaged in a close relationship with another human being.

Certain basic client-centred skills may be identified, although as we have noted, it is the total relationship that is important. Skills exercised in isolation amount to little; the warmth, genuineness and positive regard must also be present. On the other hand, if basic skills are not considered, then the counselling process will probably be shapeless or it will degenerate into the counsellor becoming prescriptive. The skill of standing back and allowing the client to find his own way is a difficult one to learn. The following interventions or skills may help in the process.

questions
reflection
selective reflection
empathy building
checking for understanding

Each of these skills can be learned. In order for that to happen, each must be tried and practised. There is a temptation to say 'I do that anyway!' when reading a description of some of these skills. The point is to notice the doing of them and to practise doing them better! Whilst counselling often shares the characteristics of everyday conversation, if it is to progress beyond that it is important that some, if not all, of the following skills are used effectively and tactfully.

Questions

Two main sorts of questions may be identified in the client-centred approach: **closed** and **open** questions. A closed question is one that elicits a 'yes', 'no' or similar one word answer; or it is one where the counsellor can anticipate an approximation of the answer, as she asks it. Examples of closed questions are as follows:

where do you live?
are you married?
are you happier now?
are you living at home?

Too many closed questions can make the counselling relationship seem like an interrogation. They also inhibit the development of the client's telling of his story and place the locus of responsibility in the relationship firmly with the client.

Open questions

Open questions are those that do not elicit a particular answer; the counsellor cannot easily anticipate what an answer will 'look like'. Examples of open questions include:

what did you do when that happened?
how did you feel then?
how are you thinking right now?
what do you feel will happen?

Open questions are ones that encourage the client to say more, to expand on their story or to go deeper. Open questions are generally preferable, in counselling, to closed ones. They encourage longer, more expansive answers and are rather more free of value judgements and interpretation than are closed questions. All the same, the counsellor has to monitor the 'slope' of intervention when using open questions. It is easy, for example, to become intrusive by asking too piercing questions, too quickly. As with all counselling interventions, the timing of the use of questions is vital.

Questions can be used in the counselling relationships for a variety of purposes. The main ones include:

1. To clarify: 'I'm sorry, did you say you are to move or did you say you're not sure?' 'What did you say then . . .?'
2. To encourage the client to talk: 'Can you say more about that?', 'What are your feelings about that?'
3. To obtain further information: 'How many children do you have?', 'What sort of work were you doing before you retired?'
4. To explore: 'What else happened . . .?', 'How did you feel then?'

ACTIVITIES FOR IMPROVING INTERPERSONAL SKILLS IN THE HEALTH PROFESSIONS Number 6.

Noticing non-verbal behaviour

Simply, notice the link, or sometimes the lack of it, between what people say and their non-verbal behaviour. Which is 'correct' - the verbal or the non-verbal? Probably the only way to find out is to ask them. Notice whether or not you are consistent in your use of non-verbal behaviour.

Other sorts of questions

There are other ways of classifying questions and some to be avoided. Examples of other sorts of questions include:

Leading questions These are questions that contain an assumption which places the client in an untenable position. The classic example of a leading question is: 'When did you stop beating your wife?' Clearly, however the question is answered, the client is in the wrong! Other examples of leading questions are:

1. Is your depression the thing that's making your work so difficult?
2. Are your family upset by your behaviour?
3. Do you think that you may be hiding something . . . even from yourself?

The later, pseudo-analytical questions are particularly awkward. What could the answer possibly be?

Value-laden questions Questions such as 'Does your homosexuality make you feel guilty?', not only poses a moral question but guarantees that the client feels difficult answering it.

Why questions These should always be used sparingly (Schulman, 1982). The 'why' question can easily sound interrogative and even moralistic. Also, to ask 'why' about how someone feels is to suggest that they may know why they feel the way they do; this is often not the case. Why questions also lead to a theoretical debate about how the person is feeling. Thus the answer to 'why do you feel depressed?' will always be an offering of that person's theory of why they are depressed. It is often far more useful to discuss the feeling itself.

Confronting questions Examples of these may include: 'Can you give me an example of when that happened?' and 'Do you still love your wife?' Confrontation in counselling is quite appropriate once the relationship has fully developed but needs to be used skilfully and appropriately. It is easy for apparent 'confrontation' to degenerate into moralizing. Heron (1986) and Schulman (1982) offer useful approaches to effective confrontation in counselling.

Reflection

Reflection (sometimes called echoing) is the process of reflecting back the last few words, or a paraphrase of the last few words, that the client has used, in order to encourage them to say more. It is as though the counsellor is echoing the client's thoughts and as though that echo serves as a prompt. It is important that the reflection does not turn into a question and this is best achieved by the counsellor making the repetition in much the same tone of voice as the client used. An example of the use of reflection is as follows:

> *Client*: We lived in Edinburgh for a number of months. Then we moved and I supposed that's when things started to go wrong . . .
>
> *Counsellor*: Things started to go wrong . . .

Used skillfully and with good timing, reflection can be an important method of helping the client. On the other hand, if it is overused or used clumsily it can appear stilted and is very noticeable. Unfortunately, it is an intervention that takes some practise and one that many people anticipate learning on counselling courses. As a result, when people return from counselling courses, their friends and relatives are often waiting for them to use the technique and may comment on the fact! This should not be a deterrent as the method remains a useful and therapeutic one.

Selective reflection

Selective reflection refers to the method of repeating back to the client a part of something they said that was emphasized in some way or which seemed to be emotionally charged. Thus selective reflection draws from the middle of the client's utterance and not from the end. An example of the use of selective reflection is as follows:

> *Client*: I had just started work. I didn't earn very much and I *hated* the job. Still, it was better than being unemployed, I suppose. It's very difficult these days . . .
> *Counsellor*: You hated the job . . .
> *Client*: It was one of the worst periods of my life. I'll never forget working there . . .

The use of selective reflection allowed the client in this example to develop further an almost throwaway remark. Often, these 'asides' are the substance of very important feelings and the counsellor can often help in the release of some of these feelings by using selective reflection to focus on them. Clearly concentration is important, in order to note the points on which to selectively reflect. Also, the counselling relationship is a flowing, evolving conversation which tends to be 'seamless'. Thus, it is little use the counsellor storing up a point which she feels would be useful to selectively reflect; by the time a break comes in the conversation, the item will probably be irrelevant! This points out, again, the need to develop 'free floating attention': the ability to allow the ebb and flow of the conversation to go where the counsellor takes it and for the counsellor to trust her own ability to choose an appropriate intervention when a break occurs.

ACTIVITIES FOR IMPROVING INTERPERSONAL SKILLS IN THE HEALTH PROFESSIONS Number 7.

Using 'trigger' films for discussion

Select pieces of films or prepare your own that illustrate a small bit of interpersonal behaviour. The clip should not be more than three or four minutes long. Use the clip or a series of them to trigger off discussion in an interpersonal skills training course.

Empathy building

This refers to the counsellor making statements to the client which indicate that she has understood the feeling that the client is experiencing. A certain intuitive ability is needed here, for often

49

empathy building statements refer more to what is implied than what is overtly said. An example of the use of empathy building statements is as follows:

> *Client*: People at the factory are the same. They're all tied up with their own friends and families . . . they don't have a lot of time for me . . . though they're friendly enough . . .
> *Counsellor*: You sound angry with them . . .
> *Client*: I suppose I am! Why don't they take a bit of time to ask me how I'm getting on? It wouldn't take much! . . .
> *Counsellor*: It sounds as though you are saying that people haven't had time for you for a long time . . .
> *Client*: They haven't. My family didn't bother much . . . I mean, they looked as though they did . . . but they didn't really . . .

The empathy building statements, used here, are ones that read between the lines. Now sometimes such reading between the lines can be completely wrong and the empathy building statement is rejected by the client. It is important, when this happens, for the counsellor to drop the approach all together and to pay more attention to listening. Inaccurate empathy building statements often indicate an overwillingness on the part of the counsellor to become 'involved' with the client's perceptual world at the expense of accurate empathy! Used skilfully, however, they help the client to disclose further and indicate to the client that they are understood.

Checking for understanding

Checking for understanding involves either a) asking the client if you have understood them correctly or b) occasionally summarizing the conversation in order to clarify what has been said. The first type of checking is useful when the client quickly covers a lot of topics and seems to be 'thinking aloud'. It can be used to further focus the conversation or as a means of ensuring that the counsellor really stays with what the client is saying. The second type of checking should be used sparingly or the counselling conversation can get to seem rather mechanical and studied. The following two examples illustrate the two uses of checking for understanding.

Example a) asking

> *Client*: I don't know what to do really . . . money's OK and I can cope at home . . . well, some of the time I can cope at home . . . then there's the job. I mean, what do you do?
>
> *Counsellor*: Let me just get things a little more clear . . . You say that you don't always cope at home and you don't cope all that well at work . . .?
>
> *Client*: Yes . . . My parents treat me as though I'm still about 14 and people at work aren't much better!

Example b) summarizing

> *Counsellor*: Let me see if I can just sum up what we've talked about this morning. We talked about your financial problems and the question of seeing the bank manager. You said you may ask him for a loan. Then you went on to say how you felt you could organize your finances better in the future . . .?
>
> *Client*: Yes, I think that covers most things . . .

Some counsellors prefer to use the second type of checking at the end of each counselling session and this may help to clarify things before the client leaves. On the other hand, there is much to be said for not 'tidying up' the end of the session in this way. If the loose ends are left, the client continues to think about the issues that have been discussed as he walks away from the session. If everything is summarized too neatly, the client may feel that the problems can be 'closed down' for a while or even worse, that they have been 'solved'! Personal problems are rarely simple enough to be summarized in a few words and the process of checking at the end of a session should be used sparingly.

These, then, are particular skills that encourage self-direction on the part of the client and can be learned and used by the counsellor. They form the basis of all good counselling and can always be returned to as a primary way of working with the client in the counselling relationship.

Learning counselling skills

Counselling skills can be developed in a variety of ways. Perhaps, for the beginner (if there is such a person) they are best learned in a small group setting such as the workshop. The essential ingredients of such a workshop, as with other sorts of interpersonal skills workshops are:

1. An adequate theoretical framework. This can be supplied by the workshop facilitator either in the form of a handout, a short lecture or, preferably, through group discussion.
2. Discrimination between different sorts of counselling intervention. The neophyte counsellor needs to be able to consciously choose between different sorts of counselling interventions. Here an analysis such as Heron's (1986) *Six Category Intervention Analysis*, can be useful. For a description of this analysis see p. 28.
3. Examples or role models of effective counselling interventions are required. These may be supplied in various ways:
   a) the workshop facilitator may model them, in front of the group, with one of the group acting as 'client';
   b) the facilitator may do a monodrama and play 'both ends' of a role-play as a demonstration of effective use of counselling interventions;
   c) short video films may be used which are exemplars to the group of effective use of interventions;
   d) the facilitator may only describe the interventions and leave the group members to improvise from the descriptions.
4. All the group members need practise in using the interventions. Initially, this practise may take place within the workshop itself. Increasingly, however, the practice should be encouraged away from the workshop setting to encourage reinforcement of the new behaviour in the 'real' situation: the client/health professional relationship.

In the final chapter of this book, a variety of counselling skills exercises are described which will help the facilitator to set up and run a counselling skills workshop. Content for the 'theory' aspect of such a workshop can be gathered from the various titles outlined in the reference section of the book.

It is asserted here that counselling skills are the basic building blocks for skilled interpersonal living. The health professional who can learn to use skillfully a range of counselling skills will find the development of the other interpersonal skills discussed here considerably easier.

ACTIVITIES FOR IMPROVING INTERPERSONAL SKILLS IN THE HEALTH PROFESSIONS Number 8.

Giving positive feedback

It is often quite easy to tell other people what annoys us about them. Try telling people you work or live with how much you appreciate what they do. This can be used (often with much hilarity) in a group context. Each member of the group says what they like or appreciate about each other member in turn.

ASSERTIVENESS

Assertiveness is often confused with being aggressive. A friend of mine once referred to assertiveness workshops as 'courses for learning how to be rude to other people!' The assertive person is the one who can state clearly and calmly what she wants to say, does not back down in the face of disagreement and, if necessary, is prepared to repeat what she has to say. A continuum may be drawn that accounts for a range of types of behaviour ranging from the submissive to the aggressive, with assertive behaviour being the mid point on such a continuum (Figure 3.1). Heron (1986) has argued that when we have to confront another person we tend to feel anxiety at the prospect. As a result of that anxiety we tend to either 'pussyfoot' (and be submissive) or 'sledgehammer' (and be aggressive); so it is with being assertive. Most people, when they are learning how to assert themselves experience anxiety and as a result tend to be either submissive or aggressive. Other people handle that anxiety by swinging right the way through the continuum. They start submissively, then develop a sort of confidence and rush into an aggressive attack on the other person. Alternatively, some people deal with their anxiety by starting an encounter very aggressively and quickly back off into submission. The level and calm approach of being assertive takes practise, nerve and confidence.

Examples of how assertiveness can be useful include the following situations:

1. when used by the client who has never been able to express her wants and needs in a marriage;
2. when used by the health professional, when facing bureaucratic processes in trying to get help for her client;
3. in everyday situations in shops, offices, restaurants and other

Fig. 3.1 A continuum of assertive and non-assertive behaviours

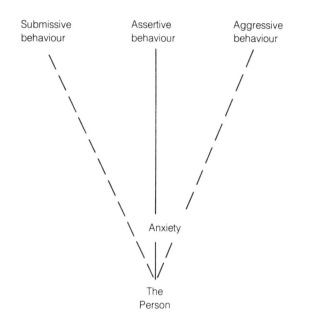

places where a stated service being offered is not actually being given.

Arguably, the assertive approach to living is the much clearer one when it comes to dealing with other human beings. The submissive person often looses friends because they come to be seen as duplicitous, sycophantic or as a 'doormat'. On the other hand, the aggressive person is rarely popular perhaps, simply, because most of us don't particularly like aggression. The assertive person comes to be seen as an 'adult' person who is able to treat other people reasonably and without recourse to either childish or loutish behaviour. Much has been written about the topic of assertiveness and the reader is referred to the recommended reading list at the end of this volume.

Alberti and Emmons (1982) identify four major elements in assertive behaviour:

1. **Intent**: the assertive person does not intend to be hurtful to others by stating his own needs and wants;
2. **Behaviour**: behaviour classified as assertive would be evaluated

by an 'objective observer' as honest, direct, expressive and non-destructive of others;

3. **Effects**: behaviour classified as assertive has the affect on the other of a direct and non-destructive message by which that person would not be hurt;

4. **Socio-cultural context**: behaviour classified as assertive is appropriate to the environment and culture in which it is demonstrated and may not necessarily be considered 'assertive' in a different socio-cultural environment.

Thus Alberti and Emmons invoke some ethical dimensions to the issue of assertiveness. They are suggesting that, used correctly, assertive behaviour is not intended to hurt the other person, should not be perceived as being hurtful and that assertive behaviour is dependent upon culture and content. They further suggest that assertive behaviour can be broken down into at least the components listed below.

Eye contact

The assertive person is able to maintain eye contact with another person to an appropriate degree.

Body posture

The degree of assertiveness that we use is illustrated through our posture, the way in which we stand in relation to another person and the degree to which we face the other person squarely and equally.

Distance

There seems to be a relationship between the distance we put between ourselves and another person and the degree of comfort and equality we feel with that person. If we feel overpowered by the other person's presence, we will tend to stand further away from them than we would do if we felt equal to them. Proximity in relation to others is culturally dependent but, in a common sense way, we can soon establish the degree to which we, as individuals, tend to stand away from others or feel comfortable near to them.

Gestures

Alberti and Emmons suggest that appropriate use of hand and arm gestures can add emphasis, openess and warmth to a message and can thus emphasize the assertive approach. Lack of appropriate hand and arm gestures can suggest lack of self-confidence and lack of spontaneity.

Facial expression/tone of voice

It is important that the assertive person is congruent in their use of facial expression (Bandler, and Grinder, 1975). Congruence is said to occur when what a person says is accompanied by an appropriate tone of voice and by appropriate facial expressions. The person who is incongruent may be perceived as unassertive. An example of this is the person who says he is angry but smiles as he says it: the result is a mixed and confusing communication.

Fluency

A person is likely to be perceived as assertive if he is fluent and smooth in his use of his voice. This may mean that those who frequently punctuate their conversation with 'ums' and 'ers' are perceived as less than assertive.

Timing

The assertive person is likely to be able to pay attention to his 'end' of a conversation. He will not excessively interrupt the other person nor will he be prone to leaving long silences between utterances.

Listening

As was noted about the effective counsellor, the assertive person is likely to be a good listener. The person who listens effectively not only has more confidence in his ability to maintain a conversation but also illustrates his interest in the other person. Being assertive should not be confused with being self-centred.

Content

Finally, it is important that what is said is appropriate to the social and cultural situation in which a conversation is taking place. Any English person who has been to America will know abut the unnerving silence that is likely to descend on a conversation if he uses words such as 'fag' or 'lavatory' in certain settings! So will the person who uses slang or swear words in inappropriate situations. It is important, in being perceived as assertive, that a person learns to use appropriate words and phrases.

A paradox emerges out of all these dimensions of assertive behaviour. The assertive person also has to be *genuine* in his presentation of self. Now if that person is too busy noticing his behaviour and verbal performance, he is likely to feel distinctly self-conscious and contrived. It would seem that assertiveness training, like other forms of interpersonal skills training tends to go through three stages and an understanding of those stages can help to resolve that paradox.

Stage one: The person is unaware of his behaviour and unaware of the possible changes that he may bring about in order to become more assertive.

Stage two: The person begins to appreciate the various aspects of assertive behaviour, practises them and temporarily becomes clumsy and self-conscious in their use.

Stage three: The person incorporates the new behaviours into his personal repertoire of behaviours and 'forgets' them, but is perceived as more assertive. The new behaviours have become a 'natural' part of the person.

It is asserted that if behaviour change in interpersonal skills training is to become relatively permanent, the person must learn to live through the rather painful second stage of the above model. Once through it, the new skills become more effective as they are incorporated into that person's everyday presentation of self.

ACTIVITIES FOR IMPROVING INTERPERSONAL SKILLS IN THE HEALTH PROFESSIONS Number 9

Attending workshops

Try to attend workshops on interpersonal skills training on a regular basis even if you are a trainer yourself. You will see other people facilitating groups and learn new ideas.

Learning to be assertive

In developing assertiveness in others, the trainer is clearly going to have to be able to role-model assertive behaviour herself. The starting point in this field, then, is personal development if it is required. This can be gained through attendance, initially, at an assertiveness training course and later through undertaking a 'training the trainers' course. There are an increasing number of colleges and extra mural departments of universities which offer such courses and they are also often included in the list of topics offered as evening courses.

Once the trainer has developed some competence in being assertive, the following stages need to be followed in the organization of a successful training course for others:

Stage One: A theory input which explains the nature of assertive behaviour, including its differentiation from submissive and aggressive behaviour.

Stage Two: A discussion of the participant's own assessment of their assertive skills or lack of them. This assessment phase may be enhanced by volunteers role-playing typical situations in which they find it difficult to be assertive.

Stage Three: Examples of assertive behaviour from which the participants may role-model. These may be offered in the form of short video film presentations, demonstrations by the facilitator with another facilitator, demonstrations by the facilitator with a participant in the workshop or through demonstrations offered by skilled people invited into the workshop to demonstrate assertive behaviour. The last option is perhaps the least attractive as too good a performance can often lead to group participants feeling deskilled. It is easy for the less confident person to feel 'I could never do that'. For this reason, too, it is important that the facilitator running the workshop does not present herself as being too assertive but allows some 'faults' to appear. A certain amount of lack of skill in the facilitator can be, paradoxically, reassuring to course participants.

Stage Four: Selection, by participants, of situations that they would like to practise in order to become more confident in being assertive. Commonly requested situations may include:

1. responding assertively to a marriage partner;
2. dealing with colleagues at work more assertively;

3. returning faulty goods to shops or returning unsatisfactory food in a restaurant;
4. not responding aggressively in a discussion;
5. being able to speak in front of a group of people or deliver a short speech.

These situations can then be rehearsed using the slow role-play method described above. At each stage of the role-play, the participants are encouraged to reflect on their performances and adopt assertive behaviour if they have slipped into being either aggressive or submissive. Sometimes, this means replaying the role-play several times.

Stage Five: Carrying the newly learned skills back into the 'real world'. Sometimes the very act of having practised being assertive is enough to encourage the person to practise being assertive away from the workshop. More frequently, however, there needs to be a follow up day or a series of follow up days in which progress, or lack of it, is discussed and further reinforcement of effective behaviour is offered.

In Chapter 8, a series of activities for encouraging the development of assertive behaviour is offered. These activities may be used throughout the type of workshop described here.

SOCIAL SKILLS

In a sense, anyone reading this book already knows what social skills are. They are those essential collection of words, behaviours, gestures and manners that go to make up effective everyday encounters with others. In the health care professions, social skills are necessary in at least the following situations:

Introducing self and others to clients or patients
Working with colleagues and other professionals
Breaking bad news
Ending relationships with clients or patients
Running small groups, case conferences, educational and therapy groups

The notion of social skills has been defined in a number of ways. Michelson *et al.* (1983) identify six main elements which they regard as making up the concept of social skills. They state that social skills:

1. are primarily acquired through learning;
2. comprise specific, discrete verbal and non-verbal behaviours;
3. entail effective, appropriate initiations and responses;
4. maximize social reinforcement from others;
5. are interactive in nature and require appropriate timing and reciprocity of specific behaviours;
6. are influenced by environmental factors such as age, sex and status of the other person.

Developing these aspects of the concept, Hargie, Saunders and Dickson (1981) argue for six separate components of social skill:

1. Socially-skilled behaviours are goal directed. In other words, the person using social skills has it in mind to effect the behaviour of another person or seeks to effect a change in a social situation.
2. Socially-skilled behaviours should be interrelated, in that they are synchronized behaviours which are employed in order to achieve a common goal. Social skills, then, do not occur in a vacuum; each person in a social encounter affects the behaviour of the other and is aware of the effect on the other. Nor can single aspects of socially skilled behaviour be considered in isolation. For example, it is quite possible to be successful at maintaining effective eye contact whilst the rest of one's 'body language' is out of synchronization with the message one is trying to convey!
3. Social skills should be appropriate to the situation in which they are being employed. Social skills, once learned, must be adapted and individualized to suit a variety of ever changing social situations.
4. Social skills are defined in terms of identifiable units of behaviour which the individual displays. There are, however, problems with this behaviourally oriented approach as Trower (1984), Heron (1977) and others have acknowledged. It can be argued, for example, that as well as studying behaviour, we should be considering the person's intentions in using certain behaviour. Merely to judge a social situation by the behaviour that is occurring is to decontextualize it. An example of this sort of analysis of chunks of behaviour cut out of its context may be seen in books such as Desmond Morris' *Manwatching* (1977). Here, Morris seeks to demonstrate the 'meaning' of certain types of

body language. It can be argued, however, that behaviour only makes sense when viewed in the context of the behavers intentions and the social situation in which the behaviour occurs.

5. Social skills can be learned. This is, perhaps, the most optimistic aspect of social skills training. In keeping with the main behavioural thrust that all behaviour is learned and can therefore be unlearned, social skills can be viewed as yet further examples of human behaviour that either a) have been faultily learned or b) have not been learned at all. A problem may arise, of course, as to what constitutes 'effective' social skills and who determines what is effective and what is not!

6. Social skills should be under the control of the individual. Thus social skills are not a repertoire of behaviours that are taught by one individual to another to be used under certain prescribed conditions, but are a tool for living, in that they can be adapted by the person to enhance their everyday effectiveness in social situations.

Examples of situations in which social skills can be used are numerous. A short list of such situations may be:

In making and receiving introductions
In initiating, maintaining and finishing a conversation
In asking something of another person
In acting assertively
In displaying appropriate emotions to other people
In conducting long and short term relationships with others

Social skills may be conveniently (if rather artificially) divided up into the use of verbal and non-verbal behaviour. Verbal behaviour can be further divided up into a variety of aspects, including:

the content of what is said,
the way in which an utterance is made and the tone of voice used,
what is intended by the speaker and
what is understood by the hearer.

These last two aspects are of vital importance. It is necessary for the listener in a social situation to try to grasp what the speaker means to convey. It is also necessary for the speaker to try to convey that meaning as clearly as possible, for we always run the risk of being misunderstood. We would do well to remember the old saying that no one who has anything important to say will risk being misunderstood! On the other hand, part of being socially skilled is also having the ability to check with a speaker that a meaning has been fully grasped (see Counselling skills, p. 50).

Non-verbal behaviour

Traditionally, in the literature on the topic (Hargie, Saunders and Dickson, 1981), non-verbal behaviour has been divided into at least the following types:

1. facial expression;
2. gesture;
3. eye contact (and also the quality of the gaze) (see Heron, 1970 for a phenomenological analysis of the gaze);
4. the use or lack of use of touch;
5. proximity between the speaker and the listener in a social relationship;
6. body posture and body position (sitting, standing etc.);
7. head nods;
8. use of paralinguistic aspects of speech ('mms', 'ahs' and other encouraging or discouraging noises).

All of these verbal and non verbal aspects of behaviour have been described and analysed in considerable detail in the literature on social skills training and above in the section on assertiveness training. The reader is also referred to the reference section of this book for further details.

Beyond the individual presentation of self that may be described through verbal and non-verbal behaviour, other elements go to make up successful socially skilled behaviour. Amongst other things, the following issues need to be addressed in any social skills training group:

1. The social context of an encounter, including such issues as the relative status of each of the people involved, the degree of friendship or hostility between them and the way in which each of them 'reads' the situation. Arguably, we all interpret social situations slightly differently. It is important that two people interacting socially reach some agreement about how each is

interpreting what is happening. An example of when this agreement has not been reached is when a social 'gaffe' occurs, through one person 'overstepping' the other's definition of the social situation.

2. The question of appropriateness of clothing and dress.
3. An appreciation of the social rules that apply in any given social situation.

ACTIVITIES FOR IMPROVING INTERPERSONAL SKILLS IN THE HEALTH PROFESSIONS Number 10

Sculpting

Ask for group members to volunteer an example of an encounter with a client that did not go well. Then allow the person who volunteers the encounter to describe it to the group. Then invite a few group members to recreate the scene and to 'freeze' their postures and non-verbal behaviours.

When all group members have had the chance to observe the 'sculpt', facilitate a discussion about it.

---

4. An awareness of how to reinforce behaviour in order for it to occur more frequently. Thus, if we want someone to know that we like what they do, we must show our appreciation for them and thus encourage them to continue to behave in that way.

Learning social skills

Social skills training may be carried out on an individual or a group basis. There is considerable value in the group approach in that group members can help each other and reinforce the effective social skills as they are developed in other people. Also, the group can develop a wide range of ideas about what is and what is not effective social skill.

There is a tendency for some health professionals to view social skills training mostly in terms of therapy (Callner and Ross, 1978; Edelstein and Eisler 1976; Falloon, Lindley, McDonald and Marks, 1977). A moment's reflection on the social skills or lack of them in fellow health professionals may well reveal a need for social skills training amongst health professionals themselves. It is possible to question, for example, the degree to which many GPs exhibit a lack of social skill when interviewing patients and the degree to which many health professionals working in hospitals give little thought to their social 'presentation of self'. It is notable that expectations of social skills are to some degree culturally determined. In North America, health professionals give considerable time to the development of social skills in their colleague and client interactions (Burnard, 1987), because a high level of social skill is expected from them. In the UK, there is a tendency to write off the American approach as shallow or insincere. It is almost as though to consider what we do and how we present ourselves to others is unnatural and rather unnecessary. It is possible, however, that many health professionals in the UK would benefit considerably from assessing their presentation of self both to their colleagues and to their clients and from spending time on enhancing this presentation.

Various stages in a social skills training programme may be identified. These stages apply whether or not the training takes place in a group context.

Stage One: Assessment of the present social skills level. In this stage, a baseline of verbal and non-verbal behaviour is established by either the trainer or the participant in training.

Stage Two: Demonstration of possible alternative behaviours. Here the trainer offers the participant a range of ways of behaving that the participant may wish to incorporate into her own repertoire. Such exemplars may be demonstrated:

1. by the trainer working on his own;
2. by the trainer co-working with another trainer in a role-play;
3. by use of a short trigger video film or by use of a longer training film;
4. by identifying, through discussion, some alternatives and through the trainer or trainers role-playing the alternatives.

Stage Three: Discussion of what needs to happen in order for the participant to adopt different social behaviour. Clearly a change of behaviour means a considerable investment on the part of the participant: ideally, the participant must *want* to change. It is arguable that social skills cannot be effective if the person does not have the intrinsic motivation necessary to effect change. If such motivation is missing, there may be short term changes in behaviour but the old pattern of behaviour will soon appear if the person is not convinced of either the need to change or the effectiveness of new behaviour.

Hopefully, of course, effective new behaviour will be self reinforcing; as the newly skilled person comes to use the new behaviour he will find that it works and thus use it again.

Stage Four: Practise in the use of new behaviours. Once the participant has seen examples of possible new behaviours, he will need plenty of opportunity to try them out in the safe atmosphere and environment of the training/classroom. A useful medium for such trying out is the role-play and psychodrama described in the previous chapter.

Stage Five: Evaluation of the new behaviour and the transfer of effective behaviour into everyday life. Evaluation can be carried out by either the participant himself, by the trainer, by the trainer and the participant together or by the group. Self and peer evaluation in social skills training may be described and implemented in the following manner:

1. The trainer prepares a behaviour repertory grid which identifies aspects of behaviour to be identified.
2. The trainer, the participant and the group focus their thoughts on the performance they have just seen and 'mark' the participant on the repertory grid sheets.
3. The participant offers to the group his own evaluation of his performance through reference to the grid.
4. The group and the trainer offer the participant feedback on his performance based on their use of the grid.
5. A discussion evolves out of the more formal aspect of the evaluation procedure with the development of ideas for improving future performances.

Once further and effective skills rehearsals or role-plays have taken place, the participant must practise the new behaviour away from the training situation and in the 'real world'. Some trainers, to enhance this transfer of skills, prefer to set the participant homework in the form of a series of tasks to be undertaken that week. Examples of such tasks may be: to initiate a conversation, to ask a member of the opposite sex to go out for a drink, to open a bank account and so on. Another way of reinforcing learning is through the use of a diary or journal in which the participant (or the group members) make notes during the week away from the group about their use or lack of use of the new skills. This journal can then form the basis of an assessment discussion at the next meeting of the social skills training group.

Facilitation skills

Consider the following situations that can be part of the health care professionals role:

1. chairing meetings and case conferences;
2. running therapy groups;
3. organizing and leading learning groups;
4. helping to set up self-help groups;
5. running support and stress-management groups.

In each of these situations the health care professional is called upon to act as a facilitator. Sometimes that facilitation is of the organizations and supportive sort, sometimes it is concerned with education and at other times it forms part of therapy. There are, however, common features that link together these different types of facilitation. It is useful if every health care professional considers her performance as a facilitator and thinks about the specific skills that are entailed. Indeed, the approach adopted by this book is one that stresses the notion of the interpersonal skills trainer as facilitator: as one who 'draws or leads out' rather than one who imparts knowledge or teaches in the traditional sense. As with social skills, counselling skills and assertiveness, the skills involved in group facilitation can be learned. Furthermore, it can be asserted that the skills involved in group facilitation are very similar to those found in counselling. In a sense, group facilitation is organized client-centred counselling in groups.

Two considerations need concern us here: the overall model of facilitation that the group facilitator adopts and the specific style that she uses when running groups. Prior to those considerations, however, are the practical and organizational aspects of group facilitation. These include thinking about:

1. The size of the group. Heron (1973) suggests the 6–12–24 rule for considering the number of people that make up a small group. He argues that 6 is the minimum number for an effective group, 12 is the optimum number and 24 is the upper limit. In the present writer's experience, however, it is quite possible to run groups larger than 24 as long as the group process is well structured and that the structure allows for all members of the group to participate.
2. The environment. There is much to be said for the 'same time,

same place' maxim for running groups. The group comes to feel comfortable in meeting at the same place and in the same room and comes to associate the room with the group. Frequent changes of venue can mean frequent adaptation on the part of the group.

3. Timing. All group meetings should start and finish on time. Any underrunning or overrunning of the group can lead to complications. If the facilitator constantly lets the group overrun and then, on one occasion finishes on time, the group will be lead to question why, on this occasion, the group has finished so abruptly. Also, most people lead fairly busy lives and it seems reasonable that they should expect the group to start promptly and finish at the stated time. The facilitator who constantly underruns in terms of time may want to consider why he finishes to early.

4. Selection of group members. Sometimes, the make-up of the group will be determined by the nature of the group. The management meeting, for example, will necessarily include some people and exclude others. When group members are selected, however, the facilitator and the initial group should carefully consider the criteria for selection and the means of selection. Some questions to consider, here, are:

   a) Should the group be made up of people of roughly the same age and status, or should there be mixing? .

   b) In the case of those designated as mentally ill, should neurotic, psychotic and psychopathic people be mixed in a group, or should separate groups be convened to suit different sorts of people? Or are the classifications irrelevant? If they are irrelevant to you, are they important to other members of your staff?

   c) Should the group be an 'open' or a 'closed' group? An open group is one that other people can join as vacancies become available. The closed group is one whose membership stays constant for the life of the group. The closed group tends to become more trusting more quickly and self disclosure tends to be greater. On the other hand, open groups are more economical to run and mean that more people get the chance to join the group than is the case with a closed group.

5. Personal experience of running groups and of being a group member. There is a strong argument for suggesting that the group facilitator should be a person with considerable experience in being a member of a variety of groups prior to running one. The person who has had experience of groups will have greater

---

ACTIVITIES FOR IMPROVING INTERPERSONAL SKILLS IN THE HEALTH PROFESSIONS Number 11

Critical incidents

Ask members of an interpersonal skills group to recall one of the following incidents:
* When you dealt with someone's emotional release ineffectually,
* When you dealt with someone's anger well,
* When you broke bad news to somebody and handled the situation adequately.

Then hold a discussion on what *behaviours* made those situations effective or not effective.

---

understanding of group processes and dynamics, is likely to have a variety of role-models from which to develop his facilitation style and will have more confidence in the process of working with groups. It is suggested that health professionals who intend to facilitate groups on a regular basis (and, of course, those who intend to run interpersonal skills groups) seriously consider attending as many types of groups as they can, including: staff meetings, therapy groups, training workshops, educational courses and so on. It seems likely, of course, that many health professionals who have reached the point in their work where they are interested in running groups will have had quite considerable experience of groups in the process of developing their professional and personal development.

Styles of group facilitation

Different sorts of groups call for different styles of facilitation. In some groups, for example, it may be important that the facilitator leads the group and makes decisions on behalf of group members. In other groups (such as therapy groups) it may or may not be appropriate for the facilitator to interpret individual members contributions to the group. Heron (1977) offers six dimensions of facilitator style which, he argues, are fairly exhaustive of possible styles of group facilitation.

1. Directive ——————— non-directive dimension
2. Interpretative ——————— non-interpretative dimension

3. Confronting   ——————   non-confronting dimension
4. Cathartic   ——————   non-cathartic dimension
5. Structuring   ——————   unstructuring dimension
6. Disclosing   ——————   non-disclosing dimension

To be **directive** in a group is to offer suggestions as to what the group may do and how it may proceed. To be **non-directive** is to offer no such advice but to allow the group to evolve of its own accord.

To be **interpretative** in a group is to offer that group an explanation of what may be happening within the group. Various 'frames' of analysis may be used for making such interpretations. For example, one facilitator may offer psychodynamic interpretations; another may offer process comments – observations about what individual members of the group appear to be doing and how the group is reacting to those individuals. To be **non-interpretative** is to offer no such interpretation but to allow the group to offer its own interpretation of what is going on in the group.

To be **confronting** in a group is to challenge either individual members or the group as a whole on any given issue. For example, the group facilitator may confront the group on its timekeeping or its apparent lack of ability to stick to an agreed agenda. To be **non-confronting** is to offer no such challenge but to encourage the group to confront itself.

To be **cathartic** in a group is to allow or encourage the free expression of feelings and emotion within that group. To be **non-cathartic** is to anticipate a potentially emotional group situation and to defuse it in some way.

To be **structuring** in a group is to offer the group a pre-arranged format for that group to use as a means of progressing. This may take the form of an agenda or it may consist of a series of exercises or activities that the group can undertake to explore a particular issue. To be **unstructuring** is to refrain from bringing structure to the group instead of allowing the group to find or create its own structure.

To be **disclosing** in a group is to readily reveal one's own thoughts and feelings to that group as a near equal member of the group. To be **non-disclosing** is to refrain from disclosing to the group.

There are times when certain sorts of facilitation will be more appropriate than others. It may be useful, for example, in a group-therapy context, to encourage the free expression of emotion and thus be cathartic in style. In a staff meeting to discuss policy, a non-cathartic style may be more appropriate. In a formal teaching situation, the group facilitator is likely to be both directive and structuring. In a sensitivity group, she may be neither.

The facilitation styles analysis has many practical uses. First, it can be used as a self-assessment tool; the group facilitator can consider the six dimensions and see at what point on each of the dimensions she considers her own style to be. For example, she may find that she is generally fairly directive when running groups, yet not interpretive. She may consider herself to be not particularly confronting and yet she allows free expression of feeling within her groups. She may use considerable structure and tend towards disclosing her feelings to her groups. In this way, she can consider ways of improving or enhancing her group facilitation practice. Second, the analysis may be used as the basis of a group facilitation training programme. The six dimensions are fairly easily explained to a learning group. The analysis may then be used as a self-assessment tool within that group and a profile drawn up which indicates general strengths and weaknesses in group facilitation across the group. Ends of dimensions which indicate particular lack of skill within group members can be identified in this way and the trainer can then use experiential methods (including role-play) to encourage the development of those skills.

The process for developing the group profile, referred to above, is as follows:

1. Each person in the learning group places a tick against the two types of facilitation styles that they feel *most* skilled in using and a cross against the two styles that they feel *least* skilled in using (see Fig. 3.2).
2. The group trainer collects all the assessment sheets from group members and draws up a 'master sheet' on a white or blackboard. This master sheet shows the distribution of markings for the group (see Fig. 3.3).
3. From the array of ticks and crosses on a master sheet there emerges a tendency for crosses to cluster against certain ends of dimensions.
4. These particular ends of dimensions are then noted and used as a basis of experiential learning activities to enhance skills development in those facilitation styles.

Third, the facilitation styles analysis may be used as a research instrument for evaluating facilitation skills within an organization,

Fig. 3.2 Self-assessment sheet for use in group facilitation training sessions.

Instructions: Place a tick against the two styles that you feel *most* competent in using and a cross against the two styles that you feel *least* competent in using in group facilitation.

	Most skilled	Least skilled
Directive		
Non-directive		
Interpretative		
Non-interpretative		
Confronting		
Non-confronting		
Cathartic		
Non-cathartic		
Structuring		
Unstructuring		
Disclosing		
Non-disclosing		

college or group. Finally, it may be used as a mental *aide memoire* for the group facilitator. She may refer to it whilst running a group and thus choose her interventions in the light of that choice. In this way she will become more precise and intentional about her group skills.

Learning group facilitation skills

Learning group facilitation skills can be enhanced in various ways.

Fig. 3.3 Example of a 'master sheet' illustrating a group profile.

	Most skilled	Least skilled
Directive	✓✓✓✓✓	✕✕
Non-directive	✓✓	✕✕
Interpretative	✓	✕✕✕✕
Non-interpretative	✓✓✓✓	✕✕
Confronting	✓	✕✕✕✕✕
Non-confronting	✓✓✓✓✓✓	
Cathartic	✓	✕✕✕✕✕✕
Non-cathartic	✓✓✓	✕
Structuring	✓✓✓✓✓✓	✕
Unstructuring	✓	✕✕✕✕
Disclosing	✓✓✓	✕✕✕✕
Non-disclosing	✓✓	✕✕✕

First, it is useful if the would-be group facilitator becomes a member of a wide range of different sorts of groups and watches the facilitation style of the various people running those groups. It is particularly useful if those groups are varied in nature, for example, a committee meeting, a therapy group, a case conference and so on. As she begins to facilitate her own groups, it is then helpful if one person whom she deems to have a particularly effective style, acts as a 'mental role-model'. In other words, she runs the group by copying the style of the preferred facilitator. After a while, the personalized facilitator style emerges and the need to copy in this way becomes less obvious. In a sense, this is what we are all doing in new situations. We are 'trying out' new roles by adopting the roles we have seen demonstrated by others.

In this chapter, various types of interpersonal skills have been explored and suggestions made for teaching them. Whilst different sorts of methods have been offered, in the end many of the methods interrelate: social skills training methods may be used for developing counselling skills, techniques used in assertiveness training may be used to enhance group facilitation skills and so on. Much will depend upon the trainer's values and beliefs, experiences in facilitating previous training groups and on the sorts of training groups she has attended as a trainee. As we have noted, in the early stages of learning to teach other people interpersonal skills there is much to be said for modelling your style of facilitation on the performance of a skilled trainer whose groups you have attended. Whilst you will not be a carbon copy of that person, the experience of trying out a particular style of facilitation will be useful. That style will become modified and personalized as you develop your skill and confidence.

4

Remembering and supervising experiential learning

In previous chapters we have considered the nature of experiential learning, experiential learning methods and some of the interpersonal skills that may be learned by the experiential approach. What is also necessary is that we as students and as professional health care workers learn to pay attention to how our skills are changing and developing. In this chapter a variety of methods of enhancing skills are discussed and particular attention is paid to two concrete and practical methods of recording and enhancing interpersonal competence: the **journal** and the **mentor** system.

GAINING EXPERIENCE IN INTERPERSONAL SKILLS

The most obvious methods of monitoring progress in interpersonal skills development have been discussed already: a) practising the skills involved and b) noticing our changing and developing reactions. The practice element often comes with the job. We are involved in interpersonal relationships everyday of our professional lives so there is plenty of time for trying out new behaviour. It has to be noted, however, that the decision to try out new interpersonal behaviour must be a conscious one. It is very easy to attend a workshop on counselling skills and to believe that a lot was gained from it. The truth is, of course, that the workshop will only have been successful if the learning gained in it is transferred to the 'real' situation. There is always a danger of an interpersonal skills workshop being an 'island' in the middle of a busy working life – something that was interesting at the time, but of little practical value. The practical value will only be evident if the transfer of learning occurs. This point is an important one for those who facilitate experiential learning workshops. They must attempt to ensure that learning is carried over into real life and does not remain within the confines of the comfortable atmosphere of the workshop. To this end, some facilitators use 'homework' as a means of reinforcing learning. Others ask workshop participants to set personal contracts with themselves to try out new learning. Others, still, have follow up days on which all the participants meet again and discuss their progress or lack of it.

The second point is a reminder about the concept of 'noticing'. Not only do we need to practise new behaviour but also to reflect on what effect it has both on ourselves and on the recipients of that behaviour. As we noted in the previous chapters, it is important to practise the skill of noticing – of having our attention rooted firmly in the present, of paying attention to ourselves and to our surroundings. As with many of these personal skills, the only way to develop the skill of noticing is to do it! Try it now and continue to notice throughout the day. If you forget and your attention wanders, slowly allow it to return and keep trying!

In summary, there are three basic requirements for 'formally' developing interpersonal competence:

1. attendance at a training course or workshop;
2. practise of new interpersonal skills in the real situation;
3. continuing ability to notice what happens to us and other people when we use interpersonal skills.

We also learn new skills incidentally through a trial and error process and we also need to monitor our progress of interpersonal growth. The two methods, alluded to above, for undertaking that monitoring – keeping a journal and using the mentor system – are now described. These methods can help us to maintain and evaluate both formal and informal learning.

KEEPING A JOURNAL

There is a growing literature on the use of self and peer assessment on the interpersonal skills field (Kilty, 1976; Burnard, 1987). With the increase in interest in experiential learning is coming the realization that those taking part in interpersonal workshops and in various forms of experiential learning need to be able to develop their own criteria for checking and evaluating their own learning (Knowles,

1975, 1978, 1980). In this section, the use of one such student-centred approach is discussed: the journal as a method of self-assessment and evaluation.

It is acknowledged that the two concepts of assessment and evaluation are inextricably linked. To assess is to identify a particular state at a particular time, usually with a view to taking action to change or modify that state. To evaluate is to place a value on a course of action, to identify the success or otherwise of something that has happened. Thus assessment is often seen as something that needs to occur at the outset of an educational encounter and evaluation something that occurs at the end. In fact, evaluation necessarily leads on to reassessment and thus to another educational encounter. In this way the journal described here can be used both as an assessment tool and as an evaluation instrument.

A modified version of the journal has been used at the School of Nursing Studies, University of Wales College of Medicine, as part of a continuous assessment procedure during the Bachelor of Nursing course, during students' psychiatric nursing secondment. It has met with varying amounts of success. After an initial period of the students feeling that they would not be able to complete the journal, a number found it particularly useful and planned to continue to use it throughout other parts of their course. Others continued to find it difficult to use and one never completed it.

The instructions for completion of the journal are simple. Participants are required to make weekly entries in a suitable book under the following headings:

Problems encountered and resolution of those problems.
Application of new skills and difficulties with them.
New skills required to be learned.
Personal growth issues/self awareness development.
Other comments.

These headings can be varied according to the needs and wants of a particular group using the journal approach. No guidelines need to be given regarding the amount that is written under each heading. To prescribe a particular number of words would be over-structuring, although it may be possible to negotiate maxima and minima with the group.

Participants are encouraged to make regular entries and this regularity tends to make the process of keeping the diary easier. Participants who try to 'catch up' and complete the whole thing in one last go tend to have difficulty in remembering what has happened and generally the process is less viable.

There are several methods of using the diary as an assessment/evaluation tool. The first is to use it as a continuous focus of discussion between the facilitator and the group in an on-going group. In this way, the participants' experience is constantly being monitored and they are able to discuss their progress or lack of it as they continue with day to day field work. The second method is to use it as a means of summative evaluation at the end of a period of field work (Scriven, 1967). In this case, the following procedure may be used:

1. Both facilitator and student sit down and individually 'brainstorm' criteria for assessing the journal. Examples of items brainstormed may be:
   a) quality of writing;
   b) clarity of expression;
   c) ability to problem-solve;
   d) level of self-disclosure, etc.
2. After this brainstorming session, both facilitator and participant identify three criteria that they wish to use for assessing the journal.
3. Each then uses those criteria to write notes on their assessment of the journal and then compare those notes.

Out of this activity comes a shared view of the journal which incorporates elements of both self and facilitator evaluation. The discussion that follows can be useful to both participants and facilitator as a means of offering further feedback on performance. This method can also be used to focus on another important communication skill, the written word. This is a particularly fruitful area if the participant is, in this case, a student or trainee in the health care field. At this stage, too, a mark for the diary can be negotiated if the journal is to form part of a continuous assessment procedure.

A third method of using the journal is as part of a weekly discussion. This can serve as a means of focusing shared problems and also as a method of disseminating new information and learning. The journal can also form the basis of a seminar group, with each member in turn taking the lead to run the group.

Probably the most democratic method of deciding upon how to use the journal is to negotiate that use with the group. This should be done prior to the journal being undertaken so that all participants are clear as to who will and who will not have access to it. Journal writing calls for a considerable degree of self-disclosure and it is important, in adult learning groups, that the participants' dignity is maintained (Jarvis, 1983).

The journal as part of a total assessment and evaluation system in an interpersonal skills training course or as part of a larger training course can be a valuable and very personal means of participants maintaining a constant check on their own learning and development. The approach can be modified in a variety of ways to reflect different emphases. For instance, the bias can be towards practical skills development, or towards self-awareness. Alternatively, participants can be encouraged to develop their own headings for the journal in order to reflect their own needs and wants.

It is interesting to consider the various levels of assessment and evaluation that take place when this method is used. First, the participants have to reflect on their experience before they write. Second, they have to convert their thoughts into words and write an entry in the journal. Third, another level of assessment occurs when the journal is discussed between other group members or in a tutorial. In this way, participants are completing part of the experiential learning cycle discussed in Chapter 1. They are also fulfilling the conditions of self-disclosure and feedback from others that Luft (1969) considers necessary for the development of self-awareness. Thus the method offers a valuable educational tool on a number of levels.

SUPERVISION AND THE MENTOR SYSTEM

In learning and developing interpersonal skills we all need help at times. Sometimes it is useful if the help regularly comes from the same person and we can develop a lasting relationship with that helper. It is here that we find the basis of the notion of mentoring. The idea of having a mentor during health care training received considerable attention in the American press (Attwood, 1979) and two writers go as far as to say that 'everyone who makes it has a mentor' (Collins and Scott, 1979). Burton (1975) notes that many of the famous American playwrights and poets revealed that they had mentors at some stage in their careers. In this country, the notion has been less written about but is gaining momentum in the health care professions as a format for developing interpersonal skills in health professionals. In Torbay Health Authority (Johns and Morris,

1988) for example, the mentor relationship has been used with considerable success in working out a new style of psychiatric nurse education.

What, then, is a mentor, why do we need them and how do we train them? A mentor is usually someone older than the student and who has considerable experience of the job for which the student is being prepared. The idea of having a mentor also usually contains the idea of continuity and of the student staying with the mentor for some time. This is in contrast to more traditional approaches to health professionals' education, where continuity with teaching staff is necessarily interrupted by field experience and where students work with a qualified person for only a short period of time. With the mentor system, trainees negotiate who their mentor will be and then stay 'allocated' to that person for the length of their training. Necessarily, then, a closer relationship is likely to develop between the mentor and student than has traditionally been the case.

Darling (1984) found in her research that there were three 'absolute requirements for a significant mentoring relationship'. These were: attraction, action and effect. In the first instance, for attraction it is deemed vital that both people respect and like each other. Arguably, as the relationship develops, a transference relationship will evolve (Burton, 1975). The term transference is usually reserved as a descriptor for the nature of the relationship which develops between a psychotherapist and her client. It signifies that the client comes to see the therapist as having personal characteristics (usually positive ones) that are reminiscent of one of the client's parents. All this normally takes place at a pre or unconscious level so the client does not readily see that this is happening. The net result is usually that the client 'idealizes' the therapist and becomes very dependent on her. One of the aims of therapy is often to help the client to try to resolve this transference relationship and thus live a less dependent and more interdependent life (Burnard, 1989). It seems likely that the relationship between student and mentor is also likely to invoke transference, particularly as the mentor is already cast in the role of 'expert' by the very nature of being a mentor at all. All this suggests that mentors should be chosen very carefully. Who should do this 'choosing' remains a question for debate!

It is possible, too that the 'attraction' could include emotional and sexual attraction. The ethical position, here, is clear – at least in theory. The relationship between mentor and student should remain a platonic one, given the tacit contract that exists between teachers, clinical staff and students. Life is rarely as simple as that, however, and the issue of how to cope with more involved relationships clearly needs addressing.

In terms of the 'action' role of the mentor, the student is likely to want to use the mentor as a role model. Again, by definition, the mentor is seen as an expert: someone who has achieved the various skills that are deemed necessary for effective practice and who is able to use and pass on those skills. In a sense, this aspect of mentoring may be equivalent to the 'sitting with Nellie' approach to training office staff in some organizations. 'Sitting with Nellie' refers to the idea of learning skills by sitting with and watching the person who has them. Clearly, though, it is to be hoped that this will not be the only way that skills are passed on. Traditionally, there has been an element of this approach in the past training policies for students. Just being with a qualified person was sometimes seen as enough to encourage and enable students to develop skills. Whether or not this was ever the case is another debatable point. A certain skill in coaching seems to be a requirement of the skilled mentor. The ability to break down skills into component parts and teach them and then have the ability to demonstrate their use with the appropriate, accompanying affect, seems to be another skill to aim for. Mentoring, it would seem, is not for the faint-hearted!

From the 'affective' point of view, the mentor needs to act in a supportive role. She should be able to encourage the student, enhance her self-confidence and teach her to be constructively critical of what she sees and does. Again this aspect of the role is likely to re-open the debate about the likelihood of a transference relationship occurring. If it does and transference does occur, it is important that the mentor will be able to cope with it. She will also need to know how to close the relationship and be skilled in 'saying goodbye'. This is unlikely to be easy because of the possible 'counter-transference' that may occur: the mentor's complicated network of feelings for the student! At best, however, the relationship may come to mirror the best aspects of the truly therapeutic relationship that the student will develop with her patients. Hopefully, then, the mentor will be able to initiate and sustain the sort of exemplary relationship that will stand as a role model for future relationships. Again, a lot is being asked of the person who acts as mentor.

If such a relationship does develop and is sustained, it is likely to be very valuable for the student and, no doubt, for the mentor. If the heart of nursing is concerned with relationships, then a close relationship between one who 'knows' and one who is learning may be useful to both and, subsequently, to the patients.

On the other hand, there are numerous problems. Because of the nature of the partnership, the student starts in a 'one down' relationship with the mentor. The mentor is necessarily in a dominant position in the relationship. It is not and cannot be a relationship of equals. Much of the recent writing on adult education has suggested that adult education should concern itself with negotiation, with shared learning and with meeting students' own perceived needs (Brookfield, 1987); the adult needs to use what they learn, as they learn it; they need to be treated as equals in a partnership that leads along a road of inquiry; they need to have their self-concept protected, as they go. Now whether such demands for equality and negotiation can exist within the constraints of the mentor/student relationship is not clear. It seems more likely that the mentor will be identified as a benign (or perhaps, not so benign) father or mother substitute. Some may find such a portrayal overdramatic, but, as we have noted, the perfectly respectable notion of transference depends upon the 'unconscious designation' of the other person as a surrogate parent.

There is also the problem of the mentor's own development. There is nothing worse than the 'guru' who feels that she has gained enlightenment and all she needs to do is to sit back and pass on pearls of wisdom to others! I write 'she': unfortunately, such guru figures are nearly always male! All of us need to continue our development and education. None of us has 'arrived'; none of us is skilled to the point where we cannot learn other skills. The mentor must be a convert, if to anything, to lifelong education (Gross, 1977; Mocker and Spear, 1982).

Lifelong education is a concept that fits in well with the notion of experiential learning. With lifelong learning the assumption is that education does not and should not end with 'formal' education. Unfortunately, the preparation of many health care professionals is such that a 'front-end' model of education and training is offered. That is to say that there is a lengthy preparation period (often of between two and six years) followed by very little further education, apart from the occasional study day. The responsibility for further and continuing education thus becomes the responsibility of the individual practitioner. This is particularly pertinent to the mentor who will be responsible for helping the newcomers to the profession. Lifelong learning commends an approach entailing personal responsibility for learning. Ronald Gross, in his introductory text *The*

Lifelong Learner sums up this approach as follows:

> This idea of self-development is the link between your life and learning. A free learner seizes the exhilarating responsibility for the growth of his or her own mind. This starts when you realise that you must decide what you will make of yourself. (Gross, 1977)

Lifelong learning is concerned with growth and development. There are echoes here of Whitehead's (1932) remark, quoted in the first chapter of this book: 'knowledge keeps no better than fish!' The lifelong learner is one who does not hoard 'dead knowledge' but appreciates the changing nature of it. What serves us well as knowledge and skill, today, will to quite an extent be out of date tomorrow. No health professional can afford to allow her knowledge and skills base to become out of date. Interestingly, the task of being a mentor can help in the process of keeping up to date, for the mentor also learns from the person for whom she is mentor.

This raises an interesting paradox. Whilst the mentor takes responsibility for overseeing the learner, she must also be constantly consulting that learner about how he or she will determine the next part of his or her learning. The mentor, in other words, should always be trying to do herself out of a job.

All of these things and no doubt plenty more, need consideration before the partnership of mentoring begins. Alternatively they could be faced as they occur, which may be the more painful way.

How can mentors be trained? Should they be trained? There is a tendency, in some quarters, to be disparaging about training in the interpersonal domain. Some prefer to think of health professionals as having 'natural' ability in their field. It would seem reasonable, however, to try to identify some of the aspects of the role that would lend themselves to training. First, the mentor will need skills in identifying learning objectives with the student. This involves skilful negotiation of the students objectives. Such negotiation takes two factors into account, 1) what the student identifies as a need and 2) what the mentor identifies as a need. Together, the two people must work out a reasonable and workable programme. Second, the mentor will need to be interpersonally competent. By this I mean that they will be able to initiate and maintain a student-centred relationship which takes full account of the possibility of transference occurring. They will be skilled as a counsellor and be prepared to set aside a regular time to talk to the student. This aspect of the role may be described as the 'befriending' aspect. Thirdly, they will need coaching skills. They will require the ability, described above, to encourage learning. This is, of course, different to the skills required of a teacher, for mentors will not be teachers in the traditional sense of that term. Students will, however, by various means, learn a great deal from them!

Finally, in this tentative list of requirements, the mentor will need skills in enabling the student to self-evaluate – both the student's skills and the nature of the mentor/student relationship. Thus the mentor will be encouraging the development of self-awareness in the student. Such awareness is likely to help the student in their subsequent relationships with patients or clients. All in all, the relationship needs to be an unselfish one on the part of the mentor.

These are two important methods of evaluating and monitoring experience. Both are non-traditional methods and both offer the health professional who is learning to develop interpersonal competence the tools to develop their awareness and to identify new learning goals.

5

Educational Principles and Curriculum Design in Experiential Learning

All educational activities are underpinned by certain philosophical beliefs about the nature of education. This chapter explores two approaches to education and offers a practical example of one approach in action. In discussing the broad principles behind the experiential learning approach and considering the work of adult educators, the reader will be able to make considerations about how to plan workshop and course programmes with, rather than for, the participants. The chapter paves the way towards a discussion of the specific skills of the facilitation of experiential workshops for interpersonal skills training.

Whilst training and educational methods in health care professions vary, many of them support a traditional notion of learning. It is worth considering for example, how much time is devoted, in your own branch of the health field, to the following aspects of interpersonal skills:

counselling
group facilitation
self-awareness
coping with client's and patient's emotional release (tears, anger, fear, embarrassment)

If they are dealt with at all, how are they covered? In the form of a lecture, a discussion or experientially?

TWO APPROACHES TO EDUCATION AND LEARNING

The approach to learning suggested in this book suggests a certain

Table 5.1 Two models of education and of the curriculum.

	Classical Curriculum	Romantic Curriculum
Focus of the educational encounter	Teacher-centred	Student-centred
Aim of the educational process	Teaching	Learning
Aims and objectives	Set by teacher	Negotiated
Content of the curriculum	Decided by teacher	Evolve out of relationship between teacher and learner
Learning methods	Didactic, lecture centred	Activity, experience based
Evaluation	Exams set by teacher or examining board	Self and peer evaluation
Nature of Knowledge	Absolutist: facts are objective	Relativist: knowledge involves personal perceptions

view of education. This view is best articulated by a series of comparisons between two types of curriculum models. The Table 5.1 offers two 'ideal types' of curriculum, the **classical** and the **romantic**. This distinction has been made by a variety of writers, including the novelist Robert Pirsig (1974) and the educationalist Dennis Lawton (1973), who use them to make comparisons between types of curricula in a similar manner to that described here.

It is suggested that the two curriculum models offer two different views of the nature of education and a closer examination of the two may help to illustrate this. The classical model is teacher or tutor-centred: the teacher is the more important figure than the learner, in that they plan and execute the programme; the teacher is the 'one who knows' and the student as 'the one who comes to learn'. The romantic model, on the other hand, is student-centred and its main aim is learning. In this model the teacher acts as a resource or as a 'facilitator of learning' (Rogers, 1983); a facilitator is not a teacher but one who helps others to learn for themselves.

The romantic model is more in keeping with the experiential learning approach discussed in this book. For that reason it is worth exploring the differences between the two curriculum approaches further. The health professional who uses a particular model for teaching interpersonal skills needs to have considered her underlying values and beliefs about education if she is to be consistent in her practice. Later on, we will explore the practical implications of some of these issues.

In the classical model, aims and objectives are predetermined by the teacher. Lessons are pre-planned independently of the students. In the romantic model, aims and objectives are negotiated with the learners; a student's needs and wants are identified and then learning sessions are developed around these.

In the classical model, teaching methods are also pre-determined by the teacher. In the romantic model they are chosen through collaboration with the learners and participation in the learning process is voluntary. There is also, usually, an accent on activity; the learner is encouraged to take an active part in her own learning process.

ACTIVITIES FOR IMPROVING INTERPERSONAL SKILLS IN THE HEALTH PROFESSIONS Number 12

Giving negative feedback

In an interpersonal skills group that is comprised of members that trust each other, try a 'round' whereby each person sits and receives comments about what other members of the group would like to change about that person. The exercise can be a good one for developing the skills of giving negative feedback tactfully and carefully.

Evaluation of learning in the classical model is by tests and examinations set by the teacher or by an outside examining board. In the romantic model both facilitators and learners engage in self and peer-evaluation (Burnard, 1987b). These approaches to evaluation enable the learner to assess her own performance and to receive feedback from both the facilitator and the other people in her learning group. In this way, she receives a 'triangulated' form of evaluation: she has three sets of perceptions of her learning, instead of one.

It may be noted that the classical model involves 'teaching from above', whilst the romantic model is more concerned with the 'education of equals' (Jarvis, 1983). In the romantic model, students and facilitator are 'fellow travellers' for, as we see in Table 5.1, the view of knowledge offered in this model is relative. There are no absolute truths or facts; the views of the world are negotiated through discussion, argument and debate. Because each person's view of the world is different, so individual people's 'knowledge' will be different. In the classical model, knowledge is not relative; there are objective facts out there in the world which are subject to apprehension by those who seek them – a view of knowledge that can be traced back to at least Plato. It is the teacher's task within this model to pass on those objective facts. In the classical model, knowledge is 'impartial' and is unchanged by the one who knows it (Peters, 1966). In the romantic model, knowledge is dynamic and ever changing and very much a part of the one who does the knowing.

A similar distinction between two approaches to education is made by Paulo Freire (1972) who described the 'banking' concept of education versus the 'problem-posing' concept. The banking concept (which Freire argues is the traditional and predominant one) involves the teacher helping to fill her students with knowledge, which is later 'cashed out', relatively unchanged, in examinations. In this model, 'more knowledge' is usually synonymous with 'better educated'. Alternatively, Freire's problem-posing approach to education is a means of education through dialogue. Facilitator and students meet and exchange ideas and experiences through critical argument and debate. Neither facilitator nor student has the 'right' answer; there is room for multiple realities – different views of the world built on different experiences of that world.

Blaney (1974) summarizes the more traditional teaching and learning relationship through reference to a variety of typical criteria, including:

1. **Authority** is assumed by the educational institution and is largely external to the learner.
2. **Objectives** are determined prior to the educational encounter, and these provide the basis for programme planning and evaluation. These objectives are consonant with the aims of the providing agency, although they may be revised by the teacher.
3. **Methods of instruction** are chosen for their demonstrated effectiveness in achieving the previously determined objectives.
4. **The teacher's roles** are those of instructional planner, manager of instruction, diagnostician, motivator and evaluator.
5. **The learner assumes** a dependent role regarding learning

objectives and evaluative criteria; the learner's task is to achieve the prescribed objectives.

6. **Evaluation** is criterion referenced, and criteria are based on the achievement of the prescribed objectives. The purpose of evaluation is to assess the effectiveness of instruction in assisting learners to achieve the prescribed objectives, to improve the programme, and to diagnose learning difficulties.

It is interesting to ponder on the degree to which education and training in the health care professions is organized within such criteria!

ADULT LEARNING

The American educator, Malcolm Knowles, has used the term **andragogy** to describe negotiated adult learning as opposed to **pedagogy** or teacher-directed child education (Knowles, 1980). Knowles argues that negotiated and experiential learning types of education are best suited to adults because:

ACTIVITIES FOR IMPROVING INTERPERSONAL SKILLS IN THE HEALTH PROFESSIONS Number 13

'New and good' exercise

Start an interpersonal skills group session off with a 'round' in which each person in turn reports something that has happened to them recently which is both 'new' and 'good'. This can be a useful and positive warmup activity.

---

1. Adults both desire and enact a tendency towards self-directedness as they mature, though they may be dependent in certain circumstances.
2. Adults' experiences are a rich resource for learning. Adults learn more effectively through experiential techniques of education such as discussion or problem-solving.
3. Adults are aware of specific learning needs generated by real life tasks or problems. Adult education programmes, therefore, should be organized around 'life application' categories and sequences according to learners' readiness to learn.

4. Adults are competency-based learners, in that they wish to apply newly acquired skills or knowledge to their immediate circumstances. Adults are, therefore, 'performance centred' in their orientation of learning. (Knowles, 1980)

All of these aspects of adult learning are appropriate in the teaching and learning of interpersonal skills in the health care professions. All professional adult people exercise a varying degree of professional autonomy. They all bring to the interpersonal learning situation a wealth of personal and occupational experience; no learners in the health professions arrive as *tabula rasa* or 'blank slates'. All health professionals, too, need to use the skills they learn for practical purposes within their lives and within their jobs. All of these aspects of adult learning are also consonant with the experiential learning approach described throughout this book, in that they emphasize the use of practical and personal experience as the keystones of learning interpersonal skills.

Knowles and Associates (1984) have identified seven components of andragogical practice that they feel are replicable in a variety of programmes and training workshops throughout the world. These components are highly relevant to the development of the experiential learning approach to interpersonal skills training, and state that facilitators must:

1. establish a physical and psychological climate conducive to learning. This is achieved physically by circular seating arrangements and psychologically by creating a climate of mutual respect among all participants, by emphasizing collaborative modes of learning, by establishing an atmosphere of mutual trust, by offering to be supportive and by emphasizing that learning is pleasant.
2. involve learners in mutual planning of methods and curriculum directions. People will make firm commitments to activities which they feel they have played a participatory, contributory role.
3. involve themselves in diagnosing their own learning needs.
4. encourage learners to formulate their own learning objectives.
5. encourage learners to identify resources and to devise strategies for using such resources to accomplish their objectives.
6. help learners to carry out their learning plans.
7. involve learners in evaluating their learning, principally through the use of qualitative evaluation modes.

Out of this discussion on the philosophical underpinnings of two approaches to the curriculum arise certain practical considerations for programme planning for health educators wishing to plan interpersonal skills courses or workshops. Brookfield (1986) discusses what he calls 'the principles of practice in community action projects'. These principles may well serve as the underlying principles for developing experiential learning workshops and training programmes for health care professionals and they underpin the principles described in this book in the discussion of experiential learning in a group setting:

1. The medium of learning and action is the small group.
2. Essential to the success of efforts is the development of collaborative solidarity among group members. This does not mean that dissension is silenced or divergence stifled; group members are able to accept conflict, secure in the knowledge that their peers regard their continued presence in the group as vital to its success.
3. The focus of the group's actions is determined after full discussion of participant's needs and full negotiation of all needs, including those of any formal 'educators' present.
4. As adults undertake the actions they have collaboratively agreed upon, they develop an awareness of their collective power. This awareness is also felt when these adults renegotiate aspects of their personal, occupational and recreational lives.
5. A successful initiative is one in which action and analysis alternate. Concentrating solely on action allows no time for the group to check its progress or alter previously agreed-upon objectives. But if the members of the group engage solely in analysis, they will never come to recognize their individuality and collective power. Empowerment is impossible without alternating action and reflection. (Brookfield, 1986)

If Knowles and Brookfield are right, adults need to use what they learn. All interpersonal learning needs to be grounded in the participants practical experience and any new learning needs to be the sort that can be applied on future occasions. Both Knowles' and Brookfield's notions of the educational principles of facilitating learning groups are entirely relevant to the running of interpersonal skills groups for health professionals, in that all learners coming to such groups (regardless of their status and regardless of the specific discipline) are adults.

In order to demonstrate these principles in action it may be useful to consider an example of an experiential learning workshop in action.

Experiential workshop on stress

It is useful to have some understanding of what an experiential learning workshop 'feels' like and how the philosophical issues discussed here can be translated into action. What follows is a description of the activities in a one day workshop. It makes extensive use of the principles of experiential learning and adult learning described in this book and acknowledges some of the problems that may arise in this sort of workshop and which are discussed in more detail in the next chapter.

The workshop is attended by 18 health professionals from various disciplines including social work, nursing, occupational therapy and physiotherapy. The workshop is led by the author and takes place in a large room in a local higher education college. The group members are sitting in a circle. Beside the facilitator is a large flip-chart pad on an easel. The workshop starts promptly at 9.00 a.m.

The facilitator introduces himself and invites members of the group to introduce themselves by stating:

1. their name;
2. their occupation
3. three other things about themselves.

These three headings are revealed on a pre-prepared flip chart sheet. The sheet with the headings is covered by a top sheet which is turned over by the facilitator as he invites the group to introduce themselves. Each member of the group then introduces themselves. Some take a little while over the task, others are faltering but fairly hasty. When each person has had a turn, the facilitator suggests that each person repeats, slowly, the name by which he or she wishes to be known. Thus the facilitator introduces himself by his first name. The round begins slowly but then speeds up and the facilitator urges the group to take time over the undertaking so that each person's name is heard by other members. This round is then followed by another slow name round. Group members are then invited to check the names of those people they are still unsure of. The facilitator checks one person's name and then other's follow suit. The ice has

91

been broken and the group looks and feels more relaxed.

Basic principles of the workshop are then spelt out. These are the voluntary principle, described above, and the proposal clause, also described. The facilitator also spells out, clearly, the timing of the workshop, giving times of coffee, tea and lunch breaks. After this he invites questions from the group; the group is clearly thawing out and beginning to talk more freely. A couple of people ask about the nature of the group and whether or not it will consist of lectures from the facilitator or whether or not it will be an 'encounter group'. The facilitator explains that the day will be activity based and allow for participants to explore their own stress and stressors and examine some practical methods of dealing with stress. These questions lead naturally to the first exercise.

The exercise is one carried out in pairs. Each pair nominates one member 'a' and one 'b'. For ten minutes 'a' talks to 'b' about 'how I react to stress'. After ten minutes, 'a' and 'b' swap roles and 'b' talks to 'a' about his or her reactions to stress. The pair are asked to note that the exercise is not a conversation. One member is only required to listen whilst the other person talks. The exercise is a type of thinking aloud.

After the exercise, which has been timed by the facilitator (who, on this occasion, is the odd man out in terms of numbers and there-fore does not take part in the exercise), the pairs are invited back into the group. They then discuss the exercise in terms of **process** and **content**. Process refers to how it felt to do the exercise; content refers to what was talked about.

The discussion is prolonged and thus forms the 'reflective' aspect of the experiential learning cycle. The facilitator could have written up the main points of the discussion, after it occurred, on one or more flip chart sheets but, on this occasion chose not to. Such deci-sions are best taken in the heat of the moment. Sometimes the *aide-memoire* is useful and the sheets can be pinned or 'bluetacked' on the wall to serve as a backcloth to the workshop. On other occa-sions, the procedure seems to get in the way of the natural flow of the group's life.

Some of the issues that come up during the two aspects of the discussion are as follows:

physical tension	difficulty with relationships
loss of concentration	panic/fear
moodiness	difficulty with sex
disinterest in work	anxiety

frustration	walking away from the situation
feeling of being overwhelmed	going off sick
loss of sleep	being judgemental of others
fatigue	angry spells
depression	etc., etc.
crying	

The facilitator then asks the group for its reactions to the results of the discussion. Theories and comments put forward by group members include:

'We all seem to experience stress differently.'
'Some aspects of stress are common to all of us.'
'I thought I was the only one who got worked up over nothing: it's a relief!'

The discussion brings the first hour and a half to a close and the group breaks for coffee, still discussing the issues involved.

On resuming, the facilitator suggests that members divide into small groups of three and four and discuss some of the causes of stress under the three headings:

1. How I cause myself stress.
2. How other people cause me stress.
3. Causes of stress within the world at large.

These headings are adapted from suggestions proposed by Bond (1986). Each group is given a flip-chart sheet and a fibre tipped pen and invited to elect a chairperson who writes down all the comments from the group. That chairperson does not edit out any suggestions but writes everything down. This is a typical brainstorming session. It is suggested that no filtering or dismissal of ideas takes place at all. In this way, the group develop freedom to think broadly and creatively. Some of the causes identified by group members are as follows:

1. How I cause myself stress

By pushing myself too hard	By not being assertive
By having too great expectations for myself	By allowing other people to walk all over me
By worrying too much	

By agreeing with everybody,
even when I don't really
By thinking about sex too much
By not getting what I want/need
By suffering from loss of
confidence/self doubt
By not thinking about my
relationships with others

By not planning my work
By allowing myself to get
depressed
By allowing others to decide
what I should do

ACTIVITIES FOR IMPROVING INTERPERSONAL SKILLS IN THE HEALTH PROFESSIONS Number 14

Guidelines for effective experiential facilitation

1. Allow plenty of time.
2. Explain the activity clearly.
3. Make sure that the 'processing' period, after the activity is twice as long as the period taken up by the activity itself.
4. Listen to participants and do not force a particular point of view on to them.
5. Make sure that all participation is voluntary.
6. Modify activities to suit this group at this time.

---

2. How other people cause me stress

By not agreeing with me
By manipulating me
By putting pressure on me to
succeed
By comparing me with other
people (particularly at work)
By not really knowing me
By getting aggressive with me
By belittling me

By being too bossy/authoritarian
By not communicating with me
By leaving me out in the cold
By not being honest with me
By being too easy with me
By doing things I don't like
By their anti-social habits
(smoking, drinking, etc.)

3. Causes of stress within the world at large

Threat of nuclear war
Violence and bombings
Child abuse
'Pressure' in general
Lack of purpose

Speed
Rise in the cost of living
Rise in the mortgage rate
Abuse of animals
Lack of housing

Lack of health care resources The government
Unemployment etc., etc.

This exercise, in groups, runs for 20 minutes after which time the facilitator invites group members to stick their charts up on the wall and to examine other people's charts as they go up. After this, there is a discussion about the process as well as the content of the exercise. The group is invited to draw conclusions (or to theorize) about what has happened. Some responses, here, include:

'I mostly create my own stress!'
'I tend to believe that everyone is stressed for most of the time.'
'I'm surprised how quickly we have got to know each other here.'
'I found the discussion of sexuality embarrassing but useful.'

This exercise is the last of the morning. As a closing activity, each person in turn is asked to state, first of all, what they liked least about the morning. They are told that they need not qualify what they say but should feel free to say anything they liked. After this round is completed, they are then encouraged to say what they liked most about the morning and again, it is suggested that they need not justify or qualify what they say. The facilitator joins in both rounds. Some of the comments from group members are illustrated below.

What I liked least about the morning . . .

the initial embarrassment;
joining in with the pairs exercises, first thing;
discussion of embarrassing subjects;
I thought things were a bit slow to start with.

What I liked most about the morning . . .

meeting new people;
comparing experience with other people;
realizing that other people feel the same as me;
pairing off;
being listened to but not judged.

Before breaking for lunch, the facilitator proposes a brief 'unfinished business' session. In this period of five minutes, group members are invited to say anything that they may be thinking or feeling, either to other group members or to the facilitator, either positive or negative. The rationale behind this activity (and this is made explicit to the group) is to raise any 'hidden agendas' and to allow further self-disclosure. It also works on the principle that it is perhaps better that things are said rather than just thought. After an initial period of silence, one person says, 'I felt quite stirred up by the discussion this morning . . . I'm surprised how easily I get worked up . . .'. Another says, 'I'm a bit annoyed that you rushed me this morning (to the facilitator) and would have preferred more time to finish what I was saying!' One member says to another, 'I enjoyed the pairs exercise with you this morning. I think we've got quite a bit in common!' After the five minutes, the group disperses and goes to lunch.

The afternoon session starts with a modified 'icebreaker'. Each person is invited to say something about themselves that they are proud of. It may be something that they have achieved or a personal quality. As usual, the facilitator takes part in the round. The round seems to recreate an atmosphere in which group members can easily talk and self-disclose.

Following this, the group brainstorms methods of relieving stress. In this activity, the facilitator acts as scribe and records the suggestions of the group on a series of flip-chart sheets. Examples of some of the methods of stress relief that are identified by the group include the following:

sleep	taking a holiday
walking/cycling/exercise	meditation
massage	yoga
drinking alcohol	having a good laugh/cry
using tranquilizers in small doses	counselling and co-counselling
having a bath	change of activity
eating	organization
smoking	discussion of relationships with
relaxation exercises	the people involved
time management	learning to be assertive
taking sick leave	etc., etc.

A discussion is then developed on the most common methods of stress relief, the ones that work and the ones that don't. As with the morning's session, there is some surprise and some relief that many people's experiences are similar.

96

The facilitator then asks the group to choose two methods from the list with which they are not particularly familiar and which they would like to try. After a brief discussion, they choose meditation and relaxation exercises. The facilitator then gives a brief theory input on the nature of relaxation exercises and on mediation. Theoretical information for such inputs has been documented by Hewitt (1977), Naranjo and Ornstein (1971), Bond (1986) and Bond and Kilty (1986).

After this the group undertakes a relaxation exercise (a script for such an activity can be found on p. 99). Following this the group reforms and discusses the process of the activity. All but one member has experienced complete relaxation. This one person has found that, paradoxically, she feels more tense through undertaking the activity and this is talked through with the group's support. After the discussion of her feelings, she feels considerably relieved and realizes that she gets most relief from stress through talking about the stressors in her life. This is useful both for her and for a number of other group members.

The facilitator now leads the group in a short meditation. The procedure for this is as follows:

1. Sit motionless, comfortably and with the eyes closed.
2. Breath quietly and gently. Breath in through the nostrils and out through the mouth.
3. Let your attention focus on your breathing.
4. Begin to count your breaths, from 1–10; 1 is the whole cycle of inhalation and exhalation, 2 is the next complete cycle.
5. When the breaths have been counted from 1–20, begin counting the next 10 and then the next and so on.
6. If you are distracted or loose count, simply return to the beginning of the process and start again.

Following the 15 minute meditation, the group are again invited to discuss what happened. This time, all members find the activity relaxing and de-stressing and remarks are made about how they were physically and mentally able to relax. A member requests details of the two activities and the facilitator offers pre-prepared handouts of them. Many say that they wish to carry on using either the relaxation script of the mediation, at other times, away from the workshop.

After tea, there is an open-ended discussion about the day's events. Participants are invited to identify the high and low spots of the day and a closing round of 'least liked' and 'most liked' is carried out. The workshop finishes on a calm but interested note and group members feel that it has been both interesting and worthwhile.

The workshop described here is just one example of how the experiential learning cycle may be put into practice. Not all the suggestions and principles suggested by Knowles and Brookfield are present in the example but a number are and the general principles of experiential and adult learning may be noted. It will also be noted that plenty of time was allowed for discussing each activity and that there was very little theory input into the day; this is in keeping with the notion of moving away from the facilitator occupying a teaching role towards a more facilitative role, as described above.

The principles illustrated in this description of one type of workshop can easily be applied to other types of courses and workshops. Taking the work of Knowles (1975) a framework for planning adult learning encounters may be developed. Such a framework includes the following stages:

1. setting the learning climate;
2. identifying learning resources;
3. running the learning group;
4. closing the group.

In the next chapter, the focus of the discussion shifts from general principles to specific examples of facilitation. Through considering her underlying educational beliefs and values and through considering the specific skills of facilitation, the health professional who teaches interpersonal skills can enhance and develop her ability and effectiveness.

ACTIVITIES FOR IMPROVING INTERPERSONAL SKILLS IN THE HEALTH PROFESSIONS Number 15

Relaxation

We communicate and work more effectively with others when we are relaxed. The following relaxation activity can be used either by the individual or with a group of people.

Lie on your back with your hands by your sides . . . stretch your legs out and have your feet about a foot apart . . . pay attention to your breathing . . . take two or three deep breaths and feel yourself begin to relax . . . now let your breathing become gentle, slow and relaxed . . . now allow your head to sink into the floor . . . your head is sinking and you feel more and more relaxed . . . allow your forehead to become smooth and relaxed . . . allow your cheeks and the rest of your face to relax . . . let your jaw relax and feel the tension easing in your temples . . . let yourself relax more and more . . . let your neck and your shoulders relax . . . now become aware of your right arm . . . let your right arm relax . . . your upper right arm . . . your lower right arm and now your right hand . . . the whole of your right arm and hand . . . completely relaxed . . . now become aware of your left arm . . . let your left arm relax . . . your upper left arm . . . your lower left arm and now your left hand . . . the whole of your left arm and hand completely relaxed . . . now allow your chest and trunk to feel heavy and relaxed . . . now your hips and pelvis and feel your seat sinking into the floor . . . now put your attention into your right leg . . . feel your right leg becoming heavy and relaxed . . . now your right foot . . . allow it to feel very heavy and very relaxed . . . now put your attention into your left leg . . . feel your left leg becoming heavy and relaxed . . . now your left foot . . . allow it to feel very heavy and very relaxed. Now notice how relaxed you feel and allow yourself a few minutes complete relaxation before you slowly sit and then stand up.

This script can be talked through to a group or can be dictated onto a tape for use by the individual. There is much to be said for the tape being prepared by the person who is going to use the tape so that they get used to hearing their own voice suggesting they relax. In this way, the injunction to relax becomes self-reinforcing.

6

Facilitating Learning Groups

INTRODUCTION

Facilitation or teaching?

As we noted in the previous chapter, the accent in the experiential
learning approach is towards the educational encounter being
student-centred rather than teacher-centred and appropriately adult-
centred. In this approach, the aim is not to initiate the group
participants into particular ways of knowing as Peters (1966) would
argue, but to encourage those people to think about their own
experience and to transform their personal knowledge and skills
through the processes of reflection, discussion and action.

Elizabeth King (1984) offers the following suggestions about the
nature of the facilitator's role:

1. They must believe students should make their own decisions and
   think for themselves.
2. They must refrain from assuming an authoritative role and adopt
   a more facilitative and listening position.
3. They must accept diversity of race, sex, values etc. amongst their
   students.
4. They must be willing to accept all viewpoints unconditionally and
   not impose their personal values on the students. The ability to
   entertain alternatives and to negotiate no-lose solutions to
   problems often leads to group decisions that are more beneficial
   for both the individual and the group.

Certain stages in the facilitation process can be described and the
facilitator needs to be aware of the process that can occur in groups.

The stages described here are modified from those offered by Malcolm Knowles (1975) in his discussion of facilitating learning groups for adults.

It is arguable that facilitation of learning has more in common with group therapy than it does with teaching. It is recommended that the person who sets out to become a group facilitator gains experience as a member of a number of different sorts of groups before leading one herself. In this way she will not only learn about group processes experientially but she will also see a number of facilitator styles. As Heron (1977) points out, in the early stages of becoming a facilitator it is often helpful to base your style on a facilitator that you have seen in action. Later, the style becomes modified in the light of your own experience and you develop your own approach.

STAGES IN THE FACILITATION PROCESS

Setting the learning climate

The first aspect of helping adults to learn is the creation of an atmosphere in which adult learners feel comfortable and thus able to learn. This is particularly important when it comes to developing interpersonal skills through experiential learning. Unlike more formal classroom learning, the experiential approach asks of the learners that they try things out, take some risks and experiment. If this is to happen at all, it needs to be undertaken in an atmosphere of mutual trust and understanding.

The first aspect of the setting of a learning climate is to ensure that the environment is appropriate. Rows of desks and chairs are reminiscent of earlier schooldays. For the adult experiential learning group it is often better and certainly more egalitarian if learners and facilitator sit together in a closed circle of chairs. Experiential learning workshops rarely involve a great deal of note taking, so desks or tables rarely serve as anything more than a barrier between learners and facilitator.

In the early stages of a workshop or learning group it is useful if the group members spend time getting to know each other. **Icebreakers** are sometimes used for this purpose. An icebreaker is a simple group activity that is designed to relax people and allow them to 'let their hair down' a little thus creating a more relaxed atmosphere, arguably more conducive to learning interpersonal skills. Three examples of icebreakers are described below.

Icebreaker One

The group stands up and group members mill around the room at will. At a signal from the facilitator, each person stops and introduces herself to the nearest person and exchanges some personal details. Each person then moves on and at a further signal, stops and greets another person in a similar way. This series of millings and pairings can continue until each group member has met every other, including the facilitator.

Icebreaker Two

A small cushion is used as this icebreaker. After each person in the group, in turn, has introduced herself by name, the cushion is thrown by the facilitator to one group member. As it is thrown, the facilitator calls out the name of the person who is receiving the cushion. That person then throws the cushion to another person and calls out that person's name. This activity carries on until all members of the group have learned the names of people in the group. The activity is a lighthearted affair and one that encourages the learning of members names through repetition.

Icebreaker Three

The group splits into pairs for five minutes. During that five minutes, each member of the pairs 'interviews' the other and finds out five or six things about them (including their name). After the five minutes, the group reforms and each person introduces the person with whom they spoke.

Other examples of icebreaking activities are described by Heron (1973), Brandes and Phillips (1984) and Burnard (1985). Their aim is to produce a relaxed atmosphere in which learning can take place, and a further gain is that they encourage group participation and the learning of names. They are used by many facilitators in the experiential learning field. Some people (including the author), however, feel more comfortable with a more straightforward form of introduction. The argument here, is that learners coming to a new learning experience are already apprehensive. Many carry with them memories of past learning experiences which may or may not have been of the 'formal' sort. To introduce those people to icebreakers too early may be to alienate them before they start. The icebreaker, by its very unorthodoxy, may surprise and upset them. A simpler form of introductory activity is to invite each person in turn to tell the rest of the group the following information:

1. their name;
2. where they work and their position in the team or organization;
3. a few details about themselves that are nothing to do with work.

It is helpful if the facilitator sets the pace for the activity by first introducing herself in this way. A precedent is thus set and the group members have some idea of both what to say and how much to say. The author recalls forgetting this principle when running a workshop in the Netherlands; as a result, each group member talked for about ten minutes apiece and what was intended to be a short introductory activity turned into a lengthy exercise! Perhaps the golden rule is to keep the activity short and sharp, and to keep the atmosphere 'light' and easy going.

Once group members have begun to get to know each other, either through the use of icebreakers or by the introductory activity described above, the facilitator should deal with 'domestic' issues regarding the group's life. These will include the following:

1. when the group will break for refreshments and meal breaks and when it will end;
2. a discussion of the aims of the group;
3. a discussion of the 'voluntary principle': that learners should decide for themselves whether or not they will take place in any given activity suggested by the facilitator and that no one should feel pressurized into taking part in any activity either by the facilitator or by the power of group pressure. It is worth pointing out that if a person find themselves to be the only person sitting out on a particular activity, they should not feel under any further obligation either (a) to take part, or (b) to justify their decision not to take part.
4. issues relating to smoking in the group when smokers are present;
5. any other issues identified by either the facilitator or by group members.

This early discussion of group 'rules' is an important part of the process of setting the learning climate. The structure engendered by this part of the day helps to allow everyone to feel part of the decision making and learning process.

Identifying learning resources

Most interpersonal skills workshops run for people in caring professions are attended by adults who have considerable life experience and work skills. They have also had considerable learning experience prior to attending such a workshop. The aim of the next stage of group development is to identify skills within the group that may serve as resources for further learning. Examples of such skills, that may be used as examples of learning models for others, may include such things as: specific counselling skills; skills with particular client groups, for example, the elderly, adolescents, people with AIDS, etc.; previous experience in groups; etc., etc.

Once such skills have been identified, they can be made use of by the group as and when opportunities arise. They can also be more formally 'written in' to the aims of the learning group by setting aside time for those people with skills to demonstrate them or through their facilitating teaching sessions with the rest of the group. It is at this stage that the facilitator needs to retain some humility. It is often difficult to appreciate, when you are running a group, that other people in that group may be more skilled than you in various respects!

Running the learning group

All that remains, once the learning climate has been established and resources within the group have been identified, is for the facilitator to establish the smooth running of the group throughout the use of various activities aimed at enhancing learning. In the last chapter of this book, a variety of exercises is offered as examples of the sorts of group activities that can be used to encourage the learning of specific interpersonal skills. Following the pattern laid down by the experiential learning cycle discussed earlier, these stages may be used in this part of the workshop:

1. brief theory input;
2. description of the exercise to be undertaken;
3. setting up of the activity with group members;
4. running of the activity;
5. discussion of group members' experiences following the activity.

Thus, for example, the first part of a workshop on counselling skills may be prefaced by a short theory input by the facilitator or by another member of the group, on the subject of listening. This input need not be a lecture but is often best treated as a fairly informal discussion, drawing on group members' experiences. Following this theory input, an exercise taken from the last chapter of this book is described to the group and instructions given as to pairing, timing and so on. The group then does the exercise. After this, two options present themselves for 'processing' the outcome of the exercise. Group members may either:

1. stay in their pairs and discuss the activity, before returning to a larger plenary session with the rest of the group, or
2. return to the group for a discussion lead by the facilitator.

Whichever format is used, the facilitator may choose to discuss either the **process** of the activity or the **content** of it. The process of an activity refers to what it felt like to undertake that activity and what learning followed as a result of those feelings. A discussion of the content is one that discusses what was talked about. In inter-personal skills training, it may be more productive to spend more time discussing the process of any given exercise than the content. In this way, group members develop the skill of noticing their own behaviour in interpersonal situations. Indeed, it is sometimes helpful to suggest that the content of pairs and small group activities remains confidential to those people taking part in the activity and that such content does not become part of the general discussion of the group. In this way, the group can quickly learn to handle true self disclosure in a safe atmosphere: a situation that closely resembles many 'real life' interpersonal encounters that the health professional will have to face.

It is useful to spend considerable time in this post-exercise discussion. Referring back to the experiential learning cycle discussed in a previous chapter, it was noted that Kolb (1984) asserts that new learning occurs when people reflect on their behaviour. The discussion following an exercise is an example of such reflection and the reflective process takes time. It should not be rushed by the facilitator nor should she attempt to suggest what outcomes the group members may have discovered through doing the exercise. It is common, in more traditional education settings, for a teacher to ask questions that begin: 'Did you notice how . . .?', or 'Most people find . . . when they do this sort of exercise.' Such questions have little relevance in this sort of educational experience. The aim is not to lead the group participants in a particular direction but to enable them to undertake the reflective process themselves and decide, for themselves, whether or not they will share their experience with other people. More useful questions, from a facilitation point of view, would be: 'What did you notice . . .?', or 'Does anyone want to talk about what they experienced during that exercise . . .?' or 'What else happened . . .?'

This is true 'facilitation' as opposed to 'teaching'. This aspect of experiential learning also points out a particular paradox: whilst the facilitator will be aiming to encourage the development of counselling, assertiveness or group skills, there is no guarantee that all group members will develop the same sorts of skills nor even that they will develop the ones that the facilitator had in mind! It is quite possible that, through the process of experiential learning, certain group members find 'different' ways of dealing with aspects of counselling or group work that had not occurred to the facilitator or that is not written up in the literature. This, perhaps, is the creative aspect of experiential learning and is in contrast to the usual type of learning that involves the passing on of previously established knowledge or skills.

Closing the group

Each facilitator will probably develop her own style of closing the group at the end of the day or at the end of a workshop. A traditional way is through summary of what the day has been about. There is an important limitation in this method, which aims at 'closure'. It is asserted that while the facilitator is summing up in this way, she is doing two things that are not particularly helpful. First, she is putting into her own words, those of the group members. Secondly, whilst she is closing in this way, group members are often, silently, closing off their thoughts about the day or the workshop in much the same way that schoolchildren begin to put their books away as soon as a teacher sums up at the end of the lesson. It may be far better to leave the session open-ended and to avoid any sort of summing up. Alternatively, rather than allowing the day or the workshop to end rather abruptly, the facilitator may chose to use one or more of the following closing and evaluating activities.

Closing activity one

Each person in turn makes a short statement about what they liked least about the day or about the workshop. Each person in turn then makes a short statement about what they liked most about the day or the workshop; no one has to justify what they say for their statement is taken as a personal evaluation of their feelings and experience.

Closing activity two

Each person in turn makes a short statement about three things that they feel they have learned during the day or the workshop. This may or may not be followed by a discussion on the day's learning.

Closing activity three

The group has an 'unfinished business' session. Group members are encouraged to share any comments they may have about the day or the workshop, either of a positive or negative nature. The rationale for this activity is that such sharing helps to avoid bottled up feelings and increases a sense of group cohesion.

Closing activity four

The group hug: group members stand in a circle and put their arms around each others shoulders to form a tightly knit circle. The group remains silent throughout this group exercise, or an agreement is made that people may be free to share any comments they may have with the group. This sort of symbolic activity may be particularly useful when self-disclosure has been high and people are feeling rather sensitive. It can help to encourage group cohesion, support and unity. Like all activities, however, it should not be a compulsory exercise: some people are naturally uncomfortable with an activity of this sort and the wise facilitator will chose this sort of activity with care.

These, then, are the stages of a typical interpersonal skills workshop and they may be adapted to suit the particular needs of the group and of the facilitator. The reader may like to refer back to the previous chapter to the example of a typical workshop and see to what degree the example there follows the stages described above.

GROUP DYNAMICS AND PROCESSES

Apart from considering the stages of group facilitation that are involved in planning a group learning session or a workshop, the facilitator also needs to know something about the dynamics or processes that can occur in such a group. The idea here, is that to be forewarned is to be forearmed! In this section, some of those processes are described and suggestions offered as to how those processes can be coped with as they occur. In the end, there can be no one way of coping with a particular process: everything is dependent upon the people concerned, the context, the perceptions of the facilitator and of group members and so on.

Pairing

Pairing in groups refers to one or other of two phenomena. First, the word can refer to two group members who talk quietly to each other, ignoring the rest of the group. It is arguable that such a manœuvre is a defensive one in that the pair are avoiding issues being discussed in the larger group by talking to each other. Pairing of this sort can be distracting to the facilitator and disruptive to the group because it means that the group is not operating as a single unit but is divided.

The second type of pairing is when two group members (and one is sometimes the facilitator) tend to discuss issues with each other, across the group, rather than sharing a 'whole group' discussion. This sort of pairing is less distracting than the previous sort but can cause problems. If the facilitator consistently pairs with another person in the group, that facilitator may tend to ignore other group members.

A variety of options are available to the facilitator for dealing with pairing when it occurs. Some of these are:

1. Ignore it and see what happens. Sometimes, pairing takes care of itself.
2. Draw attention to the fact that pairing has occurred and allow the group to resolve the issue.
3. Confront the two persons concerned. This must be done carefully if it is not to cause reminders of schooldays and bossy teachers!
4. Suggest that the group members all change seats as an 'icebreaking' activity.

5. Set a contract with the group, prior to the group's development, that all members will be on the lookout for the occurrence of such dynamics.
6. Engage one of the pair in discussion so that the pairing is at least temporarily broken up.

Scapegoating

Scapegoating is a name for the situation where one person in the group becomes the one whom the group attacks, for whatever reason. Sometimes only one or two people are involved in the attack, sometimes everyone is involved. Again, it is arguable that this is a defensive manoeuvre in that the scapegoated person becomes a focal point for the pent-up aggression of the collective group. Sometimes, the person singled out for scapegoating is a particularly strong person who is well able to cope with the hostility. At other times, a weaker member becomes the focus. The facilitator has at least the following options when scapegoating occurs:

1. stop it; this is particularly important when a weaker member of the group is under attack;
2. draw attention to its happening and allow the group to deal with it;
3. suggest a short break in the group's activities;
4. switch the discussion suddenly to another topic so as to reduce tension; usually this can only be a temporary measure;
5. ask the scapegoated person how he is feeling about what is happening and take the cue from him of what to do.

ACTIVITIES FOR IMPROVING INTERPERSONAL SKILLS IN THE HEALTH PROFESSIONS Number 16

'Hotseat' exercise

This is a group activity that can be used as an introductory activity, an 'icebreaker', for an established group or as a self-disclosure activity. Each person in the group takes it in turn to be asked questions by other members of the group about anything for three minutes. If that person does not wish to answer the question, he says 'pass'. After three minutes, the person nominates another member of the group to occupy the 'hotseat'. All members of the group, including the facilitator, takes part.

Projecting

Projection, in a group context, is where one or more of the group members identifies a mood or a quality in the group that is, in fact, a mood or a quality of that person. For example, a group member who is projecting his own anxiety may say 'I find this a very tense group', when all the other group members feel relaxed. It is clearly important to distinguish between descriptive comments about the group and examples of projections! Sometimes a group member will be offering a useful description of what is happening in the group and this should not be too readily written off as projection.

Another version of projection is when the group-as-a-whole comes to view an aspect of the world-outside-the-group in a hostile or aggressive way. For example, common group projection is the 'group moan', where members get caught up in a fairly circular discussion about how dreadful the 'organization' or 'management' is and how helpless the group is given these circumstances. Again, it is important for the facilitator to be able to distinguish between the group describing an accurate situation and a group projection.

When projection occurs, the facilitator can try one or more of the following interventions:

1. ignore it and see what happens;
2. offer the idea of projection to the group as a group 'interpretation' and see what the group does with the idea;
3. ask the group to consider what they think may be happening in the group and allow it to make its own interpretations.

League of Gentlemen

This expression was coined by John Heron (1973) and refers to a variant of pairing, whereby a small sub-group of people disrupt a group by forming a hostile and often sarcastic body of people whose aim is to make life in the group difficult. Often such a league is formed by one central and dominant figure who draws into quiet discussion, by use of sub-vocal 'asides', the member of the group sitting either side of him. It is recommended that the league of gentlemen is always dealt with fairly quickly, for otherwise its effects can be very detrimental to the life of the group. Confronting the league of gentlemen is nearly always difficult. Some suggestions of how this can be achieved include:

1. Direct confrontation: the sub-group leader is challenged about what is happening. This nearly always leads to a power struggle between the facilitator and the leader of the 'league of gentlemen'.
2. The facilitator asks the group to notice what is happening in the group and allows the 'league of gentlemen' to surface as an issue. Unfortunately, it may not!
3. The facilitator discloses her own discomfort at what is happening within the group. This intervention is often disarming to the league.

Wrecking

This is a 'one person' version of the league of gentlemen. Here, an individual member of the group, for whatever reason, attempts to sabotage the group. This can take place in a variety of ways. The person may, for instance, consistently disagree with everything the facilitator says or does. He may refuse to take part in any activities and encourage others to do the same. He may always be late in coming to the group or suddenly walk out of it. He may, on the other hand, offer non-verbal resistance by remaining silent but indicating constant displeasure by use of facial expression. Wrecking, as a group process, often occurs when people are 'sent' to interpersonal skills training groups rather than coming of their own volition. A number of interventions are available:

1. The person may be directly confronted about his behaviour. As with direct confrontation of the league of gentlemen, the confrontation is likely to be met with direct denial and a power struggle ensues between the wrecker and the facilitator.
2. The group's attention may be drawn to the fact that something is happening within the group and comments invited.
3. The facilitator may choose to talk to the person, on his own, outside of the group and try to reach an understanding of what is happening. Sometimes wrecking behaviour can be a cover for deep unhappiness or distress on the part of the wrecker. Whether or not the facilitator chooses to investigate the deeper meanings of the wrecking behaviour will depend on the facilitator's beliefs about the aims of the group and on her expertise and training in that sort of work.

Flight

Sometimes the intensity of a group becomes too much for an individual member or for the entire group. Emotions have been stirred, people are feeling threatened, it seems likely that someone will openly express emotion. At such times, it is not uncommon for the individual or the group to 'take flight'. They do this by changing the subject, injecting humour into the discussion, or by becoming silent. If the facilitator is unaware of what is happening, she may find that she, too, has taken flight, and the discussion has quickly moved away from its original subject. There are various ways of handling flight, including the following:

1. Point out to the group that it is happening and allow the group to take its own course.
2. Ignore it and see what happens.
3. Encourage it; this is to work paradoxically (Riebel, 1984). The paradoxical intervention is one that is apparently the completely wrong intervention at the right time. Thus, by encouraging the behaviour that is happening is to take a step towards changing that behaviour. An example from a therapeutic context may help here. The normal response to someone who is suffering from extreme anxiety is to help them to calm down. They may be asked to take deep breaths or to try to relax. Yet these are the very things that they cannot do! The paradoxical approach is to suggest that they become even more anxious. Very frequently, when a person is encouraged (or 'allowed') to do this, they laugh and find the anxiety beginning to drain away. Arguably what has happened is that they have been encouraged and allowed to do the very thing that they are good at doing. In the process they have found the means to reverse their problem; so it is with encouraging flight in a group. As the group is encouraged to change tack or to laugh so they quickly come to acknowledge what they have been doing. It is usually not long before someone in the group picks up the fact that the group has been running away from itself.

   The paradoxical approach to working with groups and interpersonal skills training workshops is an interesting and varied one. The method of encouraging a group activity that you want to change is always an option (Heron, 1986; Fay, 1978).
4. Gently bring the group or the individual back on track and away from the flight. It is useful to go back and discuss what has happened.

Shutting down

This is a particular sort of internal flight that can occur when an individual in a group is threatened by what is happening to that group. When a person shuts down, they become silent and withdrawn and appear to be taking little interest in what is going on in the group. Shutting down usually only occurs in groups where emotions are running high or where 'hidden agenda' (see below) have been suddenly made explicit. The shut down person needs gentle handling and some of the options are:

1. Offering simple, physical support, if the person is sitting next to the facilitator. If the facilitator reaches out and merely touches the person or holds their hand or arm, it can help the person to feel acknowledged. It may also trigger off the release of pent-up emotion and the person may begin to cry. In this case it is often helpful if the facilitator can allow the emotion and thus enable the shut down person to gently 'thaw out'.
2. Verbally acknowledging that the facilitator is aware of the shut down person. Here the facilitator allows the person to express some of the things that they are feeling. Again, pent-up emotion may be expressed.
3. Moving on to new topics. If the shut down person is finding the group heavy going, it is sometimes kinder to change the subject that is under discussion to a more emotionally neutral one. Arguably, however, this is merely to put off the time when the issues that have caused the person to become shut down, are discussed.
4. Asking the group to support the shut down person. Here, the group is made aware that one of its members is cutting himself off from the group's activities and the group is asked for suggestions for helping that person. This intervention, if it is used badly, can slip rapidly into group patronage!

Rescuing

Rescuing is the opposite of scapegoating. Here, a member of the group is always being protected by one or more other members of the group. Sometimes, the person being rescued sets themselves up to be rescued. They may, for example, offer to the group a presentation of self which says 'I can't cope and need help'. Clearly, too, a degree of rescuing is reasonable in that we all need to be helped out sometimes when the going gets rough. On the other hand, persistent rescuing disallows the person being rescued the chance to make decisions for himself or to find ways of coping with difficult situations within the group. In the health care professions, there are often a number of people who are 'compulsive carers' and who always want everything to work out well. When a group contains a number of such people, it is usually inevitable that considerable rescuing will take place. The facilitator can use at least one or more of the following interventions when rescuing occurs:

1. ignore it and see what happens;
2. ask the person being rescued what he would like to do;
3. confront the rescuer directly;
4. consult the group about what they think is going on in the group;
5. ask the person being rescued to speak for himself.

Hidden agenda

In all groups, at least two things are happening: the group is following an overt or obvious agenda – the activities that they are engaged in. At another level, however, all sorts of hidden or undisclosed 'agenda' are being played out. These are the issues and problems that group members bring to the group that lay outside the main or overt agenda. Kilty (1987) makes a useful set of distinctions between three sorts of hidden agenda that are frequently at work in an interpersonal skills learning group: work agenda; interpersonal agenda; personal agenda. **Work agenda** are those concerned with perceived competence and relationships at work. The person who is hiding an agenda about work may be thinking, as they sit in the group 'What do my colleagues think of my performance so far?' or 'have I damaged my reputation at work?'

Interpersonal agenda are concerned with rivalries, competition, conflicts and so forth. The person who is working from an interpersonal hidden agenda may be wondering 'Does the group leader still like me?', or 'do people in this group think themselves more intelligent than me?' and so forth. Personal agenda are to do with the individual's own concerns about themselves and their lives. The person who is working with a personal agenda may be wondering 'can I cope with the emotional intensity of this group?', or 'will I get very upset if I take part in this role-play . . . and then, what will happen?'

Hidden agenda affect the life of the group in that issues from such agenda are 'playing in the background' of the life of the group at all times. Sometimes, too, they emerge and become part of the regular or overt agenda. For example, when two group members disagree in a group discussion, the hidden agenda may emerge when one says to the other 'That's typical . . . you always thought you were better than me, anyway . . . you're always like that at work!' Here, the issue is no longer confined to what is happening in the group but has become an issue of personal disagreement and disharmony that may have been simmering in the background for days, months or years and has suddenly become explicit. When hidden agenda become overt in this way, the facilitator has at least two options:

1. to allow the hidden agenda issue to play itself out between the members of the group;
2. to invite the group to explore the hidden agenda that is emerging.

The first option is the 'softer' one and may be useful when there is neither time nor a contract with the group to explore personal issues. The second option is the more confronting and needs to be handled tactfully and non-judgementally by the facilitator and by the rest of the group.

In a mature group (either in terms of age or of experience) an interesting (and confronting) practice is to explore the hidden agendas that are lurking beneath the surface. One means of doing this is to invite group members to pair off and to verbalize, in those pairs, what they perceive to be the hidden agenda that they bring to the group. Such an activity can be rewarding in terms of the growth of the group but it is not recommended for the faint-hearted! Even if group members do not make explicit all of the hidden agenda that they bring to the group, the very act of taking part in the pairs activity will bring those agenda nearer to the surface.

All of these group processes commonly occur in groups of all sorts. They are, perhaps, more common in therapy and self awareness groups but also crop up in learning groups. A useful way of exploring such processes is to use an exercise which involves the ground rules indicated below. A discussion held using these ground rules will often enhance the development of group processes and will also make them more noticeable to the group. After the discussion has been run for about an hour using the rules, they can be dropped and a discussion encouraged about what happened. The ground rules can also be adopted on a regular basis as a means of enhancing clear and assertive communication between group participants.

Ground rules for a group discussion

1. Say 'I', rather than 'you', 'we' or 'people' when discussing. Rather than 'people in this group are getting a bit edgy', say 'I am getting a bit edgy'.
2. Speak directly to other people rather than speaking about them. For example, rather than 'I think what John is saying is . . .', say 'John, you seem to me to be saying that . . .'.
3. Avoid theorizing about what is happening in the group. Theorizing can often lead to a dry 'academic' discussion and can lead the group away from discussing how they are feeling as the group unfolds.
4. Try to stay in the present tense: discuss what you are thinking and feeling now.

Gendlin and Beebe (1968) offer another set of ground rules which may either be used as an alternative to the ones already cited, or they may be used alongside them. These ground rules have a broader application than the previous ones and are not value-free: they presuppose a particular view of groups. It is interesting to ponder on the degree to which you agree with their use in a health care/ interpersonal skills training context.

1. everyone who is here belongs here just because he is here and for no other reason;
2. for each person what is true is determined by what is in him, what he directly feels and finds making sense in himself and the way he lives inside himself;
3. our first purpose is to make contact with each other – everything else we might want or need comes second;
4. we try to be as honest as possible and to express ourselves as we really are and really feel – just as much as we can;
5. we listen to the person inside – living and feeling;
6. we listen to everybody;
7. the group leader is responsible for two things only; he protects the belonging of every member and he protects their being heard if this is getting lost;
8. realism: if we know things are a certain way, we do not pretend they are not that way;

9. what we say here is 'confidential': no one will repeat anything said here outside the group, unless it concerns only himself. This applies not just to obviously private things, but to everything. After all, if the individual concerned wants others to know something, he can always tell them himself;
10. decisions made by the group need everyone taking part in some way;
11. new members become members because they walk in and remain – whoever is here belongs.

It is interesting to reflect on the degree to which you could use this set of ground rules in your own area of training. It is sometimes helpful to negotiate this second set of rules with the particular group and then such ground rules can serve as a group contract – to be adhered to by all group members for the life of the group.

SELF AND PEER EVALUATION

At the end of any learning encounter it is usual to undertake an appraisal in order to plan future learning sessions. The concept of self and peer evaluation has been alluded to in the discussion about both philosophical and practical aspects of experiential learning. Such an approach offers learners the chance to consider their own skills and learning and also to offer feedback on skills and learning to others. The approach is easily described and is best broken down into stages.

1. The learning group 'brainstorms' criteria for evaluation. These may or may not include such things as:
   (a) contribution to the group;
   (b) degree of self-awareness shown;
   (c) level of self disclosure
   etc., etc.
2. The list of criteria generated by the brainstorming session is prioritized and the first five criteria are selected as those suitable for use in the evaluation activity.
3. Each person in the group (including the facilitator) spends ten minutes on her own, considering her performance and levels of learning under the headings of the five criteria.
4. The group reforms and one person outlines their evaluation of themselves to the group.

5. That person then receives both negative and positive feedback from the group, under the five headings. This is the 'peer' element of the activity and is, like all other activities, voluntarily entered into. Some people may prefer not to receive peer feedback.
6. Once one person has undergone the self and peer review, the process moves onto the next person in the group and the cycle is repeated: first the individual offers the group her appraisal and evaluation, then the group offers feedback. As we have noted, the facilitator enters the evaluation process as an equal and does not necessarily have the first or the last word.

This process of self and peer evaluation takes time. Performed properly, with a group of about 10 people, it can occupy a whole afternoon and can be a valuable means of developing self-awareness and of forward planning for future learning activities. It may be used either as a form of formative evaluation or as a form of summative evaluation (Scriven, 1967). That is to say that it can be used in the middle of a course as a means of judging progress or it can be used at the end of a course as a method of deciding on the effectiveness and usefulness of the course.

This chapter has taken a practical look at the processes involved in facilitating interpersonal skills groups. It has considered that process in stages, from the opening of the group to the final evaluation. It has also discussed some of the processes and dynamics that can occur in such groups and has offered two sets of ground rules for use in interpersonal skills work. The next stage in the process of learning about experiential learning in interpersonal skills development is to try it out! The next chapter describes how the exercises offered in the final chapter may be used.

7

Using Experiential Learning Activities

This chapter offers concrete guidance on the use of the exercises for interpersonal skills development offered in the final chapter. Each exercise is laid out under a series of headings, as follows:

Aim of the activity

Here, the intention of the activity is made clear. What can never be written for such exercises is a series of behavioural objectives. As we have noted throughout this book, experiential learning is necessarily idiosyncratic. It is not possible to predict the outcome of a particular exercise for any particular person. All that can be said is that there is a clear intention in setting out to offer the exercise as a learning activity.

Number of participants recommended

Whilst a minimum and maximum figure is quoted for each activity, many of the activities can be adapted for larger numbers. Many, too, can be carried out by only two persons, learning as a pair. If larger numbers are being catered for, it is important that a great deal of structure is used in organizing the exercise. In groups of 20 and above, it is helpful if the instructions for the activity are written out in the form of a pre-prepared handout, so that everyone is clear about how to proceed. It is also helpful if, during the feedback and processing session, the larger group is broken up into smaller groups of about four or five people. Many do not like discussing their experience in a large group and constraints of time may mean that not everyone gets heard in a larger group. A chairperson may be nominated or elected in each feedback group. A short plenary session with the whole group may be facilitated afterwards as a means of maintaining group cohesion.

Environmental considerations

The usual suggestion, here, is that group members sit round in a circle. Such a circle is symbolic of unity and also ensures that the group facilitator is on an equal footing with the group and not physically (and symbolically) set apart from it. It is important, too, that the group does not sit around a table or in front of desks. In this way, there are no physical barriers between participants. The arrangement also allows for greater ease of movement if the exercise calls for the group's splitting into pairs or smaller groups.

Equipment required

None of the exercises calls for equipment which is difficult to obtain. The most important feature of the exercises is the personal one: the meeting of people to enhance their skills.

Time required

Taking time over these activities is very important. None of them should be rushed and plenty of time should be allowed for the discussional part of the activity.

The activity

This section, in each case, offers a clear stage by stage account of how to run the exercise. Initially it is useful if these instructions are followed to the letter. Once the facilitator and the group have become familiar with the approach, various modifications can be made to suit the circumstances. Many of the most effective activities are those that the facilitator devises herself. On the other hand, as was noted above, it is important that none of the exercises is rushed.

Evaluation procedure

This section offers clear guidelines as to how to encourage the group to reflect on its learning. Again, the process should not be foreshortened nor hurried.

When to use the exercises

The activities described in the following chapter can be used as they stand in workshops and other forms of interpersonal skills training. Combined with icebreaker or other introductory exercises, they can form the basis of an entire programme on aspects of interpersonal skills. They can also be combined with more didactic sessions that consider theoretical and research aspects of interpersonal skills. Such theory inputs, it is suggested, should be kept short so as to avoid the more traditional 'teacher centred' approach predominating. I have found that a theory input can often be offered in the form of a handout with headings, that can serve as a discussional document. References to further reading can also be supplied in this manner.

Questions: pitfalls and problems

Activities in groups are always different to the way they are described in books. No two groups are the same and what suits one group of people may not suit another. There are bound to be uncertainties about procedure and about group activity on the part of both the facilitator and group members. It is often this 'uncertainty' element that makes groups interesting and a powerful source of learning. In the closing section of this chapter, various questions are posed about experiential learning activities and group procedure. They are ones frequently asked in training groups for facilitators and a variety of possible solutions is offered for each one.

What happens if the learners don't want to join in?

It is important that all of these activities are entered into voluntarily. No one should be forced to undertake an activity against their will. If a relaxed and informal atmosphere is maintained, most people will find the activities useful and interesting.

What happens if no one says anything during the discussional period?

This is where the use of a flip-chart pad or blackboard can help. If the facilitator is clearly prepared to make notes on what happens, then people's contributions to a discussion are seen to be valued. However, the use of such jotting down can sometimes serve to break up the discussion and in some cases this approach should be abandoned in favour of free discussion. The keyword here is flexibility. It is important that the facilitator listens to what the group wants and needs and modifies the programme and the activities to suit that group.

What if one person talks too much in a discussion?

The facilitator has a number of options here:

1. she can allow the person to carry on overtalking and allow the group to deal with the issue;
2. she can 'shut out' the person gently by holding up her hand and by drawing in other members of the group;
3. she can raise the issue of contributions made by group members with the group and allow the issue of the dominant person to emerge;
4. she can directly confront the person and gently indicate that he is overtalking.

What if someone gets emotional during an exercise?

Sometimes some experiential learning activities generate emotion. Again, the facilitator has a number of options available to her:

1. She can make a contract with the group, at the beginning of the session, to the effect that the expression of emotion is 'allowed' or even that it may be encouraged. This option is best used by someone who has had training in coping with emotional release. Courses on coping with cathartic release are offered by a growing number of colleges and extra-mural departments of universities.
2. She can note the developing emotional involvement and can switch the topic of conversation to a lighter note, so that emotional release is avoided.
3. She can acknowledge both to the individual and to the group, that

emotions are rising and can ask the individual and/or the group what they wish to happen.

What if the facilitator feels that things are getting out of control?

This issue is usually linked to the previous one and relates to emotional expression by one or more members of the group. A simple method of coping with this is to 'lighten' the atmosphere with a change of activity or a change of pace. Alternatively, the facilitator can suggest that the group takes a short break and that everybody be allowed a 'cooling off' period.

What happens if the group falls silent?

This issue is considered in one of the exercises in group facilitation. Invariably there will be periods of silence in a group workshop. Sometimes the silence 'feels' uncomfortable and is a necessary lull in the proceedings. At other times the silence feels hostile and it is helpful if the facilitator can confront the silence and invite the group to offer thoughts about why the silence has occurred or perhaps to invite questions about any 'hidden agenda' that may be at work in the group. Also, the silence may indicate a natural pause in the proceedings, signalling time for a change of activity or a break. Finally, a silence can indicate a loss of direction by the facilitator, by the group, or both. Sometimes it can be helpful to disclose that you are lost in such circumstances; self-disclosure at times such as these can indicate that like all other members of the group, you are human and need help at times.

What happens if someone walks out of the group?

Again, there can be many reasons for a person leaving the group unannounced: tension; embarrassment; heightened emotion; boredom; hostility; a forgotten appointment; and so forth. It is helpful if a decision is made prior to starting a learning group about whether or not people should be free to leave when they choose. If the agreement is that people can leave, then nothing, normally, need be done if someone walks out. On the other hand, if the agreement is that no one leaves without indicating their intention to do so, it may be helpful to send someone to talk to the person who absences themselves without warning. It is rarely helpful for the facilitator to leave the group to speak to the person who walks out. On the other hand, there will always be exceptions to these guidelines: unusual situations call for unusual interventions!

Can the activities be used in groups smaller in number than six?

Generally the activities described here require a reasonably sized group (between 6 and 24) to enable the experiential learning cycle to be fully worked through. On the other hand, a number of the activities, including those concerned with counselling, assertiveness and social skills, can be carried out in pairs. If they are carried out between two people, it is important to stick to the structure of the activity and allow plenty of time for discussion of the activity after it has finished.

Does interpersonal skills training have to be all experiential learning?

No, ring the changes: the occasional formal lecture to fill in background information or to deepen group participants' thinking about a certain aspect of interpersonal relations can be very useful. On the other hand, lecturing can be seductive! It can be tempting and easy to slip back into the traditional 'information-giving' mode of the teacher or lecturer. Sometimes it is far more difficult to remain a facilitator than it is to return to a more familiar approach to teaching and learning. The pull is often in two directions, (a) the group seems to be asking for information and for a lecture, and (b) it seems appropriate to 'give in' and hand out information. It is often helpful to discuss this occurrence with the group as it happens rather than just slip back into information-giving.

Do I have to be trained in using experiential learning methods?

Experience in a variety of group situations is an advantage when using experiential learning activities. Experience of this sort can be gained in a number of ways. First, the would-be facilitator can take part in as many different types of group as possible, as a member. This will allow her to study other people's facilitation style and to observe group dynamics and how they are dealt with. Secondly, a number of colleges and extra-mural departments of universities offer short workshops on facilitating groups. These tend to run either for one or two days, or for a full week. Thirdly, more formal training can be undertaken via enrolment of a part or full-time course in group work. Again, such courses are offered by various colleges and universities and also by certain organizations specializing in particular sorts of group therapy, for example Gestalt, Psychodynamic or Analytical therapies. Such courses are usually advertised in health service journals and in journals about groups and about psychotherapy. I have found a balance between formal training, attending occasional workshops and informally finding out as I go along a useful way to proceed. Again, it is a question of lifelong and experiential learning. No one ever stops learning about groups and group facilitation.

The final chapter of this book offers a range of exercises for interpersonal skills training. The exercises have all been used by the author in a variety of contexts and always with health care professionals. They are representative of a wide range of activities for encouraging the development of interpersonal skills, using the experiential learning approach, but are clearly not exhaustive of all possible types of exercises that can be used. More can be found in the items contained in the further reading list at the end of the book. I have found the experiential way of working interesting, rewarding and always surprising. I have found that the exercises here work and I hope that you will too; good luck!

8

Experiential Learning Activities for Health Professionals

ACTIVITIES FOR DEVELOPING COUNSELLING SKILLS

Activity number one

Aim of the Activity: to explore not listening to another person.

Number of participants recommended: between 5 and 25.

Environmental considerations:
Participants should start the exercise by sitting in a circle, in a large well lit and well ventilated room. There should be enough space for people to be able to move around in and within which to move their chairs. Alternatively, a series of smaller rooms can be used.

Equipment required: a flip-chart pad, white or blackboard and marking pen or chalk.

Time required: 45 minutes to 1 hour.

The activity:
The group breaks up into pairs and the pairs move to various parts of the room so that they are not immediately overheard by other pairs. In each pair, one person is nominated A and the other B. A then talks to B for five minutes about any subject, while B does *not* listen to them! After five minutes, roles are reversed and A sits whilst B talks and A does not listen.

After a second five minutes, the group reconvenes and group members discuss what it was like not to be listened to. These comments may be jotted down onto a flip-chart sheet, white or blackboard, by the facilitator.

Evaluation procedure:
At the end of the activity each member, in turn, is asked to say two things that they learned from the activity. They are then invited to say (a) what they liked least about it, and (b) what they liked most about it. Alternatively, participants may be invited to write down their thoughts about the activity, for their own use.

Activity number two

Aim of the activity: to explore listening to another person.

Number of participants recommended: between 5 and 25.

Environmental considerations:
Participants should start the exercise by sitting in a circle, in a large well lit and well ventilated room. There should be enough space for people to be able to move around in and within which to move their chairs. Alternatively, a series of smaller rooms can be used.

Equipment required: a flip-chart pad, white or blackboard and marking pen or chalk.

Time required: 45 minutes to 1 hours.

The activity:
The group breaks up into pairs and the pairs move to various parts of the room so that they are not immediately overheard by other pairs. In each pair, one person is nominated A and the other B. A then talks to B for five minutes about any subject, while B *listens* to them! After five minutes, roles are reversed and A sits whilst B talks and A listens. It is important that the pairs are told that this activity is not a conversation and that the partners' role is one of listening only.

After a second five minutes, the group reconvenes and group members discuss what it was like not to be listened to. These comments may be jotted down by the facilitator.

Evaluation procedure:
At the end of the activity each member, in turn, is asked to say two things that they learned from the activity. They are then invited to say (a) what they liked least about it, and (b) what they liked most

about it. Alternatively, participants may be invited to write down their thoughts about the activity, for their own use.

Activity number three

Aim of the activity: to practise **noticing**.

Number of participants recommended: between 5 and 25.

Environmental considerations:
Participants should start the exercise by sitting in a circle, in a large well lit and well ventilated room. There should be enough space for people to be able to move around in and within which to move their chairs. Alternatively, a series of smaller rooms can be used.

Equipment required: a flip-chart pad, white or blackboard and marking pen or chalk.

Time required: 45 minutes to 1 hour.

The activity:
The concept of noticing, as described in the text of this book, is related to group members. The group breaks up into pairs and the pairs move to various parts of the room so that they are not immediately overheard by other pairs. In each pair, one person is nominated A and the other B. A then talks to B for five minutes about any subject, while B listens to them and practises noticing, as the other person talks. B should be instructed to notice everything that is going on, both inside herself and in the environment immediately in front of her. After five minutes the roles are reversed and A sits whilst B talks and A listens and notices.

After a second five minutes, the group reconvenes and group members discuss what it was like to be listened to. These comments may be jotted down by the facilitator.

Evaluation procedure:
At the end of the activity each member, in turn, is asked to say two things that they learned from the activity. They are then invited to say (a) what they liked least about it, and (b) what they liked most about it. Alternatively, participants may be invited to write down their thoughts about the activity, for their own use.

Activity number four

Aim of the activity: to practise asking questions of another person.

Number of participants recommended: between 5 and 25.

Environmental considerations:
Participants should start the exercise by sitting in a circle, in a large well lit and well ventilated room. There should be enough space for people to be able to move around in and within which to move their chairs. Alternatively, a series of smaller rooms can be used.

Equipment required: a flip-chart pad, white or blackboard and marking pen or chalk.

Time required: 45 minutes to 1 hour.

The activity:
The group breaks up into pairs and the pairs move to various parts of the room so that they are not immediately overheard by other pairs. In each pair, one person is nominated A and the other B. A then asks open and closed questions of B about any subject, while B listens to those answers but does not allow the exercise to become a conversation. After five minutes, roles are reversed and B asks open and closed questions of A.

After a second five minutes, the group reconvenes and group members discuss what happened during the exercise. These comments may be jotted down by the facilitator.

Evaluation procedure:
At the end of the activity each member, in turn, is asked to say two things that they learned from the activity. They are then invited to say (a) what they liked least about it, and (b) what they liked most about it. Alternatively, participants may be invited to write down their thoughts about the activity, for their own use.

Activity number five

Aim of the activity: to practise the use of **reflection**.

Number of participants recommended: between 5 and 25.

129

Environmental considerations:
Participants should start the exercise by sitting in a circle, in a large well lit and well ventilated room. There should be enough space for people to be able to move around in and within which to move their chairs. Alternatively, a series of smaller rooms can be used.

Equipment required: a flip-chart pad, white or blackboard and marking pen or chalk.

Time required: 45 minutes to 1 hour.

The activity:
The group breaks up into pairs and the pairs move to various parts of the room so that they are not immediately overheard by other pairs. In each pair, one person is nominated A and the other B. A then talks to B for ten minutes about any subject, while B practises the use of reflection. After ten minutes, roles are reversed.

After a second ten minutes, the group reconvenes and group members discuss what happened during the activity. These comments may be jotted down by the facilitator.

Evaluation procedure:
At the end of the activity each member, in turn, is asked to say two things that they learned from the activity. They are then invited to say (a) what they liked least about it, and (b) what they liked most about it. Alternatively, participants may be invited to write down their thoughts about the activity, for their own use.

Activity number six

Aim of the activity: to practise a combination of facilitative interventions.

Number of participants recommended: between 5 and 25.

Environmental considerations:
Participants should start the exercise by sitting in a circle, in a large well lit and well ventilated room. There should be enough space for people to be able to move around in and within which to move their chairs. Alternatively, a series of smaller rooms can be used.

Equipment required: a flip-chart pad, white or blackboard and marking pen or chalk.

Time required: 45 minutes to 1 hour.

The activity:
The group breaks up into pairs and the pairs move to various parts of the room so that they are not immediately overheard by other pairs. In each pair, one person is nominated A and the other B. A then initiates a conversation with B and uses *only* facilitative interventions (open questions, closed questions, reflections or empathy building statements) during that conversation. After ten minutes, roles are reversed and B initiates a conversation with A, using only facilitative interventions during that conversation.

After a second ten minutes, the group reconvenes and group members discuss what happened during the activity. These comments may be jotted down by the facilitator.

Evaluation procedure:
At the end of the activity each member, in turn, is asked to say two things that they learned from the activity. They are then invited to say (a) what they liked least about it, and (b) what they liked most about it. Alternatively, participants may be invited to write down their thoughts about the activity, for their own use.

Activity number seven

Aim of the activity: to explore bad counselling.

Number of participants recommended: between 5 and 25.

Environmental considerations:
Participants should start the exercise by sitting in a circle, in a large well lit and well ventilated room. There should be enough space for people to be able to move around in and within which to move their chairs. Alternatively, a series of smaller rooms can be used.

Equipment required: a flip-chart pad, white or blackboard and marking pen or chalk.

Time required: 45 minutes to 1 hour.

The activity:

The group breaks up into pairs and the pairs move to various parts of the room so that they are not immediately overheard by other pairs. In each pair, one person is nominated A and the other B. A spends ten minutes using a range of counselling skills *as badly as possible*! After this ten minutes, roles are reversed and B counsels A, using counselling skills as badly as possible. The aim in each case should be to demonstrate how counselling should not be practised.

After a second ten minutes, the group reconvenes and group members discuss what happened during the activity. These comments may be jotted down by the facilitator.

Evaluation procedure:

At the end of the activity each member, in turn, is asked to say two things that they learned from the activity. They are then invited to say (a) what they liked least about it, and (b) what they liked most about it. Alternatively, participants may be invited to write down their thoughts about the activity, for their own use.

Activity number eight

Aim of the activity: to identify personal counselling skills.

Number of participants recommended: between 5 and 25.

Environmental considerations:

Participants should start the exercise by sitting in a circle, in a large well lit and well ventilated room. There should be enough space for people to be able to move around in and within which to move their chairs. Alternatively, a series of smaller rooms can be used.

Equipment required: a flip-chart pad, white or blackboard and marking pen or chalk.

Time required: 45 minutes to 1 hour.

The activity:

The group breaks up into pairs and the pairs move to various parts of the room so that they are not immediately overheard by other pairs. In each pair, one person is nominated A and the other B. They then spend ten minutes identifying what they consider are their strengths and weaknesses as counsellors. Each person, in each pair, invites another person to assess her strengths and weakness as well as undertaking a personal assessment.

After ten minutes, the group reconvenes and group members discuss what happened during the activity. These comments may be jotted down by the facilitator. The items identified during this activity may then be used as the basis of a counselling skills workshop.

Evaluation procedure:
At the end of the activity each member, in turn, is asked to say two things that they learned from the activity. They are then invited to say (a) what they liked least about it, and (b) what they liked most about it. Alternatively, participants may be invited to write down their thoughts about the activity, for their own use.

Activity number nine

Aim of the activity: to practise introductions and closure in a counselling session.

Number of participants recommended: between 5 and 25.

Environmental considerations:
Participants should start the exercise by sitting in a circle, in a large well lit and well ventilated room. There should be enough space for people to be able to move around in and within which to move their chairs. Alternatively, a series of smaller rooms can be used.

Equipment required: a flip-chart pad, white or blackboard and marking pen or chalk.

Time required: 45 minutes to 1 hour.

The activity:
The group breaks up into pairs and the pairs move to various parts of the room so that they are not immediately overheard by other pairs. In each pair, one person is nominated A and the other B. A then practises opening a counselling session with B. Participants should be encouraged to explore a wide range of expressions,

133

phrases and approaches in order to discover what suits them and what does not. A then practises closing the counselling session, again spending time practising a wide range of possibilities. After ten minutes, A and B swap roles and B practises openings and closings with A.

After ten minutes, the group reconvenes and group members discuss what happened during the activity. These comments may be jotted down by the facilitator.

Evaluation procedure:
At the end of the activity each member, in turn, is asked to say two things that they learned from the activity. They are then invited to say (a) what they liked least about it, and (b) what they liked most about it. Alternatively, participants may be invited to write down their thoughts about the activity, for their own use.

Activity number ten

Aim of the activity: exploring silence.

Number of participants recommended: between 5 and 25.

Environmental considerations:
Participants should start the exercise by sitting in a circle, in a large well lit and well ventilated room. There should be enough space for people to be able to move around in and within which to move their chairs. Alternatively, a series of smaller rooms can be used.

Equipment required: a flip-chart pad, white or blackboard and marking pen or chalk.

Time required: 45 minutes to 1 hour.

The activity:
The group breaks up into pairs and the pairs move to various parts of the room so that they are not immediately overheard by other pairs. In each pair, one person is nominated A and the other B. Each pair then spends ten minutes sitting facing each other in total silence. Each person is encouraged to reflect on how they feel about the silence and to note what physical and behavioural manifestations the silence brings about.

After ten minutes, the group reconvenes and group members discuss what happened during the activity. These comments may be jotted down by the facilitator.

Evaluation procedure:
At the end of the activity each member, in turn, is asked to say two things that they learned from the activity. They are then invited to say (a) what they liked least about it, and (b) what they liked most about it. Alternatively, participants may be invited to write down their thoughts about the activity, for their own use.

ACTIVITIES FOR DEVELOPING ASSERTIVENESS

Activity number eleven

Aim of the activity: to explore aspects of assertiveness.

Number of participants recommended: between 5 and 25.

Environmental considerations:
Participants should start the exercise by sitting in a circle, in a large well lit and well ventilated room. There should be enough space for people to be able to move around in and within which to move their chairs. Alternatively, a series of smaller rooms can be used.

Equipment required: a flip-chart pad, white or blackboard and marking pen or chalk.

Time required: 45 minutes to 1 hour.

The activity:
The group breaks up into pairs and the pairs move to various parts of the room so that they are not immediately overheard by other pairs. In each pair, one person is nominated A and the other B. A then sits opposite B and says 'yes' to them; B replies 'no'. The pairs are encouraged to explore the use of these two words with various tones and volumes of voice. The activity must not involve conversation, but only the words yes and no. After five minutes, roles are reversed and A says 'no' to B's 'yes'.

After a second five minutes, the group reconvenes and group members discuss what happened during the activity. These comments may be jotted down by the facilitator. The group also explores how individual members cope with saying 'no' to other people.

Evaluation procedure:
At the end of the activity each member, in turn, is asked to say two things that they learned from the activity. They are then invited to say (a) what they liked least about it, and (b) what they liked most about it. Alternatively, participants may be invited to write down their thoughts about the activity, for their own use.

Activity number twelve

Aim of the activity: to explore aspects of assertiveness.

Number of participants recommended: between 5 and 25.

Environmental considerations:
Participants should start the exercise by sitting in a circle, in a large well lit and well ventilated room. There should be enough space for people to be able to move around in and within which to move their chairs. Alternatively, a series of smaller rooms can be used.

Equipment required: a flip-chart pad, white or blackboard and marking pen or chalk.

Time required: 45 minutes to 1 hour.

The activity:
The group breaks up into pairs and the pairs move to various parts of the room so that they are not immediately overheard by other pairs. In each pair, one person is nominated A and the other B. A then sits opposite B and says 'I want to' to them; B replies 'you can't'. The pairs are encouraged to explore the use of these two phrases with various tones and volumes of voice. The activity must not involve conversation, but only the two phrases. After five minutes, roles are reversed and A says 'you can't' to B's 'I want to'.

After a second five minutes, the group reconvenes and group members discuss what happened during the activity. These comments may be jotted down by the facilitator.

Evaluation procedure:
At the end of the activity each member, in turn, is asked to say two things that they learned from the activity. They are then invited to say (a) what they liked least about it, and (b) what they liked most about it. Alternatively, participants may be invited to write down their thoughts about the activity, for their own use.

Activity number thirteen

Aim of the activity: to practise giving bad news.

Number of participants recommended: between 5 and 25.

Environmental considerations:
Participants should start the exercise by sitting in a circle, in a large well lit and well ventilated room. There should be enough space for people to be able to move around in and within which to move their chairs. Alternatively, a series of smaller rooms can be used.

Equipment required: a flip-chart pad, white or blackboard and marking pen or chalk.

Time required: 45 minutes to 1 hour.

The activity:
The group breaks up into pairs and the pairs move to various parts of the room so that they are not immediately overheard by other pairs. In each pair, one person is nominated A and the other B. A then practises giving bad news to B, who responds according to the way they experience the news being given. A should bear in mind the following three stages of breaking bad news:

1. a warning that bad news is coming, followed immediately by:
2. the bad news, itself, broken clearly and calmly followed by:
3. the teller of the news offering practical support.

Examples of 'bad news' that can be broken, include: the death of a relative; the news that the person's job has had to be terminated; failure of an examination. After ten minutes, roles are reversed and B breaks bad news to A.

After a second ten minutes, the group reconvenes and group

members discuss what happened during the activity. These comments may be jotted down by the facilitator.

Evaluation procedure:
At the end of the activity each member, in turn, is asked to say two things that they learned from the activity. They are then invited to say (a) what they liked least about it, and (b) what they liked most about it. Alternatively, participants may be invited to write down their thoughts about the activity, for their own use.

Activity number fourteen

Aim of the activity: identify your style.

Number of participants recommended: between 5 and 25.

Environmental considerations:
Participants should start the exercise by sitting in a circle, in a large well lit and well ventilated room. There should be enough space for people to be able to move around in and within which to move their chairs. Alternatively, a series of smaller rooms can be used.

Equipment required: a flip-chart pad, white or blackboard and marking pen or chalk.

Time required: 45 minutes to 1 hour.

The activity:
The group breaks up into pairs and the pairs move to various parts of the room so that they are not immediately overheard by other pairs. In each pair, one person is nominated A and the other B. Each pair then spends ten minutes identifying what they consider are their strengths and weaknesses in terms of being assertive or being submissive. Each pair identifies those situations that they can handle assertively and those situations that they cannot.

After ten minutes, the group reconvenes and group members discuss what happened during the activity. These comments may be jotted down by the facilitator. The items identified during this activity may then be used as a basis of an assertiveness skills workshop. Role-play can be used to practise an assertive approach in those situations that most group members find difficult.

Evaluation procedure:
At the end of the activity each member, in turn, is asked to say two things that they learned from the activity. They are then invited to say (a) what they liked least about it, and (b) what they liked most about it. Alternatively, participants may be invited to write down their thoughts about the activity, for their own use.

Activity number fifteen

Aim of the activity: to explore assertive behaviour through slow role-play.

Number of participants recommended: between 5 and 25.

Environmental considerations:
Participants should start the exercise by sitting in a circle, in a large well lit and well ventilated room. There should be enough space for people to be able to move around in and within which to move their chairs. Alternatively, a series of smaller rooms can be used.

Equipment required: no special equipment is required for this activity.

Time required: 45 minutes to 1 hour.

The activity:
The facilitator helps the group to identify a situation which most group members would find difficult to handle in terms of being assertive. She then sets up a role-play to explore the use of an assertive approach and group members are encouraged to act out the role play with the central character practising assertive behaviour. The role-play should take place *slowly* and may be stopped at any time either by the central character or by other players in the role-play. It is stopped in order that a particular aspect may be 'replayed' and thus improved upon. The aim is to slowly build up a scenario in which assertive behaviour is demonstrated smoothly and effectively. This exercise can be compared to rehearsing a play.

Evaluation procedure:
At the end of the activity each member, in turn, is asked to say two things that they learned from the activity. They are then invited to

say (a) what they liked least about it, and (b) what they liked most about it. Alternatively, participants may be invited to write down their thoughts about the activity, for their own use.

Activity number sixteen

Aim of the activity: to explore assertiveness in a group context.

Number of participants recommended: between 5 and 25.

Environmental considerations:
Participants should start the exercise by sitting in a circle, in a large well lit and well ventilated room. There should be enough space for people to be able to move around in and within which to move their chairs. Alternatively, a series of smaller rooms can be used.

Equipment required: a flip-chart pad, white or blackboard and marking pen or chalk.

Time required: 45 minutes to 1 hour.

The activity:
The group remains in the circle and one person is invited to describe a situation in which they would like to have been assertive and were not. The person then describes the dialogue that occurred right up to the point when they failed to be assertive, for example,

'A friend asked me to go to the theatre and I didn't really want to go. I thought I would tell him that I didn't want to and promised to go on another occasion. He then said he would be very disappointed if I didn't go, so I said . . .'

Having stopped at this point, each person in the group is invited to offer an assertive response, in their own words. In this way a whole variety of perceived assertive statements is generated. When each person has made a statement in response to the suggested scenario, the person who offered the scenario is invited to suggest which of the alternatives she feels would best have dealt with the situation.

Evaluation procedure:
At the end of the activity each member, in turn, is asked to say two

things that they learned from the activity. They are then invited to say (a) what they liked least about it, and (b) what they liked most about it. Alternatively, participants may be invited to write down their thoughts about the activity, for their own use.

Activity number seventeen

Aim of the activity: to explore psychodrama.

Number of participants recommended: between 5 and 25.

Environmental considerations:
Participants should start the exercise by sitting in a circle, in a large well lit and well ventilated room. There should be enough space for people to be able to move around in and within which to move their chairs. Alternatively, a series of smaller rooms can be used.

Equipment required: various 'props' are required to make the psychodrama effective. These will become apparent as a scenario is discussed.

Time required: 45 minutes to 1 hour.

The activity:
A member of the group is invited to recall a situation in which they would like to have been assertive but were not. She then describes the whole scenario to the group in some detail and identifies the other characters that were involved in the scenario.

The person then invites other members of the group to play the parts of the other characters involved in the original scenario. The scenario is then played out as it occurred with occasional 'direction' from the person who suggested the scenario.

After this literal run through, the group stops to discuss in what ways the person could have been more assertive in the playing out. A second run through then occurs. This time, the central player relives the scene but incorporates into her action the suggestions as to how she might be more assertive. In this way, the original scenario is replayed as an assertive scenario.

After this second run through, the group then discusses to what degree the 'assertive performance' was effective.

Evaluation procedure:

At the end of the activity each member, in turn, is asked to say two things that they learned from the activity. They are then invited to say (a) what they liked least about it, and (b) what they liked most about it. Alternatively, participants may be invited to write down their thoughts about the activity, for their own use.

Activity number eighteen

Aim of the activity: to identify the behaviours that are associated with being assertive, being submissive and being aggressive.

Number of participants recommended: between 5 and 25.

Environmental considerations:

Participants should start the exercise by sitting in a circle, in a large well lit and well ventilated room. There should be enough space for people to be able to move around in and within which to move their chairs. Alternatively, a series of smaller rooms can be used.

Equipment required: a flip-chart pad, white or blackboard and marking pen or chalk.

Time required: 45 minutes to 1 hour.

The activity:

The group breaks up into pairs and the pairs move to various parts of the room so that they are not immediately overheard by other pairs. In each pair, one person is nominated A and the other B. Each pair is then given flip-chart sheets and asked to sketch caricatures of three people:

1. a submissive person;
2. an assertive person;
3. an aggressive person.

After ten minutes, the group reconvenes and group members discuss what happened during the activity. The pairs pin up their sketches and other group members are encouraged to view these. Out of this viewing of the sketches can arise a discussion about the specific behaviours that are associated with the three different sorts of behaviours. These can be listed on flip-chart sheets by the facilitator.

NOTE It is helpful (particularly for the less than artistic!) if the group members are encouraged to draw large 'matchstick men' to serve as outlines for their 'people'. In this way, facial expressions and arm and leg positions can be drawn quite easily.

Evaluation procedure:
At the end of the activity each member, in turn, is asked to say two things that they learned from the activity. They are then invited to say (a) what they liked least about it, and (b) what they liked most about it. Alternatively, participants may be invited to write down their thoughts about the activity, for their own use.

Activity number nineteen

Aim of the activity: to explore being assertive.

Number of participants recommended: between 5 and 25.

Environmental considerations:
Participants should start the exercise by sitting in a circle, in a large well lit and well ventilated room. There should be enough space for people to be able to move around in and within which to move their chairs. Alternatively, a series of smaller rooms can be used.

Equipment required: a flip-chart pad, white or blackboard and marking pen or chalk.

Time required: 45 minutes to 1 hour.

The activity:
The group is simply asked to negotiate part of the day's (or week's) proceedings. The only 'ground rule' is that they should do this assertively and ensure that their needs and wants are catered for.

Following this period of negotiation, the group members are encouraged to discuss to what degree they felt they were: submissive; assertive; or aggressive.

Evaluation procedure:
At the end of the activity each member, in turn, is asked to say two

things that they learned from the activity. They are then invited to say (a) what they liked least about it, and (b) what they liked most about it. Alternatively, participants may be invited to write down their thoughts about the activity, for their own use.

Activity number twenty

Aim of the activity: to set personal contracts.

Number of participants recommended: between 5 and 25.

Environmental considerations:
Participants should start the exercise by sitting in a circle, in a large well lit and well ventilated room. There should be enough space for people to be able to move around in and within which to move their chairs. Alternatively, a series of smaller rooms can be used.

Equipment required: a flip-chart pad, white or blackboard and marking pen or chalk.

Time required: 45 minutes to 1 hour.

The activity:
The group breaks up into pairs and the pairs move to various parts of the room so that they are not immediately overheard by other pairs. In each pair, one person is nominated A and the other B. A then writes down a number of 'resolutions' that will serve as personal reminders about how she will be more assertive in the future. She then discusses these with her partner. After ten minutes, roles are swapped and B writes down her resolutions and discusses them with A. The following format is a useful one for noting these resolutions:

Situation in which I will be more assertive	What I will have to do to be more assertive in that situation	Possible constraints
1. (e.g. Saying 'No to colleagues and friends')	(e.g. Control my anxiety; be prepared to repeat myself etc.)	(e.g. Certain friends will push me to say 'yes'; some people may not like me as a result).
2.		
3.		
4.		

After ten minutes, the group reconvenes and group members discuss what happened during the activity. These comments may be jotted down by the facilitator. Group members are encouraged to talk through their resolutions with the group and to discuss the consequences of such resolutions.

Evaluation procedure:
At the end of the activity each member, in turn, is asked to say two things that they learned from the activity. They are then invited to say (a) what they liked least about it, and (b) what they liked most about it. Alternatively, participants may be invited to write down their thoughts about the activity, for their own use.

ACTIVITIES FOR DEVELOPING SOCIAL SKILLS

Activity number twenty-one.

Aim of the activity: assessment of strengths and weaknesses.

Number of participants recommended: between 5 and 25.

Environmental considerations:
Participants should start the exercise by sitting in a circle, in a large

145

well lit and well ventilated room. There should be enough space for people to be able to move around in and within which to move their chairs. Alternatively, a series of smaller rooms can be used.

Equipment required: a flip-chart pad, white or blackboard and marking pen or chalk.

Time required: 2–3 hours.

The activity:
Group members are encouraged to 'brainstorm' activities that they feel represent awkward or difficult ones in terms of social skills. Examples, here, may be: entering a large room that is full of strangers; initiating a conversation at a party; introducing self to a stranger. Having negotiated a short list of problem situations, group members are invited to jot down that list.

The group breaks up into pairs and the pairs move to various parts of the room so that they are not immediately overheard by other pairs. Each pair then spends ten minutes identifying what they consider are their strengths and weaknesses in those situations. Group members are encouraged to identify the specific behaviours that they would or would not find difficult to use.

After ten minutes, the group reconvenes and group members discuss what happened during the activity. These comments may be jotted down by the facilitator. The items identified during this activity may then be used as the basis of a series of role-plays to practise the social skills that may be useful in these settings.

Evaluation procedure:
At the end of the activity each member, in turn, is asked to say two things that they learned from the activity. They are then invited to say (a) what they liked least about it, and (b) what they liked most about it. Alternatively, participants may be invited to write down their thoughts about the activity, for their own use.

Activity number twenty-two

Aim of the activity: exploring poor social skills.

Number of participants recommended: between 5 and 25.

Environmental considerations:
Participants should start the exercise by sitting in a circle, in a large well lit and well ventilated room. There should be enough space for people to be able to move around in and within which to move their chairs. Alternatively, a series of smaller rooms can be used.

Equipment required: a flip-chart pad, white or blackboard and marking pen or chalk.

Time required: 1–2 hours.

The activity:
The group identifies a social situation that most people would find difficult to cope with. A role-play is then set up to explore this situation and the 'actors' in the role-play are invited to play their parts by demonstrating a total lack of social skills! This can be a dramatic method of identifying, paradoxically, the social skills that are required in a given situation. It can also highlight the sorts of everyday social skills problems that occur. In exaggerating poor social skills, 'normal' and everyday presentations of self are often highlighted.

After the role-play the group reconvenes and group members discuss what happened during the activity. These comments may be jotted down by the facilitator. The items identified during this activity may then be used to practise 'proper' social skills.

Evaluation procedure:
At the end of the activity each member, in turn, is asked to say two things that they learned from the activity. They are then invited to say (a) what they liked least about it, and (b) what they liked most about it. Alternatively, participants may be invited to write down their thoughts about the activity, for their own use.

Activity number twenty-three

Aim of the activity: to assess other people's social skill levels.

Number of participants recommended: between 5 and 25.

Environmental considerations:
Participants should start the exercise by sitting in a circle, in a large

147

well lit and well ventilated room. There should be enough space for people to be able to move around in and within which to move their chairs. Alternatively, a series of smaller rooms can be used.

Equipment required: a flip-chart pad, white or blackboard and marking pen or chalk.

Time required: 45 minutes to 1 hour.

The activity:
The group breaks up into pairs and the pairs move to various parts of the room so that they are not immediately overheard by other pairs. In each pair, one person is nominated A and the other B. A then tells B what she considers to be that person's particular social skills. For example, she may say: 'I think that you handle group situations very well . . . you are particularly good at putting people at their ease . . .' and so forth. After ten minutes, roles are reversed and B then tells A what she considers to be that person's particular social skills.

After ten minutes, the group reconvenes and group members discuss what happened during the activity. These comments may be jotted down by the facilitator. Out of this discussion can emerge the areas of social skills training for further work. This exercise is best carried out only with a group that is fairly mature and whose members know each other fairly well.

Evaluation procedure:
At the end of the activity each member, in turn, is asked to say two things that they learned from the activity. They are then invited to say (a) what they liked least about it, and (b) what they liked most about it. Alternatively, participants may be invited to write down their thoughts about the activity, for their own use.

Activity number twenty-four

Aim of the activity: exploring critical incidents.

Number of participants recommended: between 5 and 25.

Environmental considerations:
Participants should start the exercise by sitting in a circle, in a large

well lit and well ventilated room. There should be enough space for people to be able to move around in and within which to move their chairs. Alternatively, a series of smaller rooms can be used.

Equipment required: a pre-prepared series of slides or a pre-prepared video film; a flip-chart pad, white or blackboard and marking pen or chalk.

Time required: 2–3 hours.

The activity:
Group members are shown either:

1. a series of slides, or
2. a short sequence of video film.

Each slide or sequence of film should graphically illustrate a difficult social situation. Examples for use, here, are:

a person pushing into a queue of other people;
a person who 'overtalks' in a conversation and doesn't allow the other person to leave the encounter;
someone making an unwelcome sexual advance.

Where slides are used, the facilitator may have to 'talk through' the action represented in the slide. The aim of both slides or video tape should be that the situations act as 'triggers' for discussion. After seeing each 'trigger', the group discusses ways that the social situation could best be dealt with. After that, a series of role-plays are set up and enacted to explore the various possibilities raised in the group discussion.

Evaluation procedure:
At the end of the activity each member, in turn, is asked to say two things that they learned from the activity. They are then invited to say (a) what they liked least about it, and (b) what they liked most about it. Alternatively, participants may be invited to write down their thoughts about the activity, for their own use.

Activity number twenty-five

Aim of the activity: trying out new body language.

Number of participants recommended: between 5 and 25.

Environmental considerations:
Participants should start the exercise by sitting in a circle, in a large well lit and well ventilated room. There should be enough space for people to be able to move around in and within which to move their chairs. Alternatively, a series of smaller rooms can be used.

Equipment required: a flip-chart pad, white or blackboard and marking pen or chalk.

Time required: 45 minutes to 1 hour.

The activity:
Participants break into pairs and spend ten minutes 'rearranging' the way each other is sitting. The person who is being arranged should remain completely flexible and allow themselves to be moved into other positions. After ten minutes the pairs return to the larger group but each person remains in the new position and a discussion is held about the nature of body language.

Evaluation procedure:
At the end of the activity each member, in turn, is asked to say two things that they learned from the activity. They are then invited to say (a) what they liked least about it, and (b) what they liked most about it. Alternatively, participants may be invited to write down their thoughts about the activity, for their own use.

Activity number twenty-six

Aim of the activity: to explore the use of eye contact.

Number of participants recommended: between 5 and 25.

Environmental considerations:
Participants should start the exercise by sitting in a circle, in a large well lit and well ventilated room. There should be enough space for

150

people to be able to move around in and within which to move their chairs. Alternatively, a series of smaller rooms can be used.

Equipment required: a flip-chart pad, white or blackboard and marking pen or chalk.

Time required: 45 minutes to 1 hour.

The activity:
The group breaks up into pairs and the pairs move to various parts of the room so that they are not immediately overheard by other pairs. In each pair, one person is nominated A and the other B. A then talks to B, whilst B listens and makes constant and sustained eye contact! After ten minutes, roles are reversed. Neither aspect of the pairs' activity should evolve into a conversation. In the 'listening' role, the person just listens and makes sustained eye contact.

After ten minutes, the group reconvenes and group members discuss what happened during the activity. These comments may be jotted down by the facilitator. The group then discusses the uses and abuses of eye contact in therapeutic and everyday situations.

Evaluation procedure:
At the end of the activity each member, in turn, is asked to say two things that they learned from the activity. They are then invited to say (a) what they liked least about it, and (b) what they liked most about it. Alternatively, participants may be invited to write down their thoughts about the activity, for their own use.

Activity number twenty-seven

Aim of the activity: to explore body posture, whilst listening.

Number of participants recommended: between 5 and 25.

Environmental considerations:
Participants should start the exercise by sitting in a circle, in a large well lit and well ventilated room. There should be enough space for people to be able to move around in and within which to move their chairs. Alternatively, a series of smaller rooms can be used.

Equipment required: a flip-chart pad, white or blackboard and marking pen or chalk.

Time required: 1–2 hours.

The activity:
Gerard Egan (1986) suggests that the following behaviours are usefully demonstrated whilst listening to another person in a therapeutic encounter:

1. sit squarely in relation to the other person;
2. maintain an 'open' position, with legs uncrossed and arms unfolded;
3. lean slightly towards the other person;
4. maintain reasonable eye contact;
5. relax.

The group breaks up into pairs and the pairs move to various parts of the room so that they are not immediately overheard by other pairs. In each pair, one person is nominated A and the other B. A then talks to B for ten minutes whilst B listens but contradicts the first four behaviours identified above. Thus, B sits next to A, she crosses her legs and folds her arms, she leans away from the other person and she maintains no eye contact with the other person. After ten minutes, roles are reversed and B talks to A whilst A contradicts the first four behaviours outlined above.

After a further ten minutes, the group reconvenes and group members discuss what happened during the activity. These comments may be jotted down by the facilitator.

In the second stage of the activity, the whole process is repeated but this time each 'listener' in the pairs adopts the listening behaviours outlined by Egan. In the discussion that follows, Egan's behaviours are discussed as to their degree of appropriateness and effectiveness in therapeutic situations.

Evaluation procedure:
At the end of the activity each member, in turn, is asked to say two things that they learned from the activity. They are then invited to say (a) what they liked least about it, and (b) what they liked most about it. Alternatively, participants may be invited to write down their thoughts about the activity, for their own use.

ACTIVITIES FOR DEVELOPING FACILITATION SKILLS

Activity number twenty-eight

Aim of the activity: to experience an absence of facilitation.

Number of participants recommended: between 5 and 25.

Environmental considerations: participants should start the exercise by sitting in a circle, in a large well lit and well ventilated room.

Equipment required: a flip-chart pad, white or blackboard and marking pen or chalk.

Time required: 45 minutes to 1 hour.

The activity:
The group activity is simple to instigate if not to carry out! Group members remain in a circle and are told that there will be no facilitator for the session (about 45 minutes) and no subject for discussion. The group is left to its own devices.

After the 45 minutes has elapsed, group members and facilitator share their perceptions of the activity.

Evaluation procedure:
At the end of the activity each member, in turn, is asked to say two things that they learned from the activity. They are then invited to say (a) what they liked least about it, and (b) what they liked most about it. Alternatively, participants may be invited to write down their thoughts about the activity, for their own use.

Activity number twenty-nine

Aim of the activity: to explore a directive style of group facilitation.

Number of participants recommended: between 5 and 25.

Environmental considerations: participants should start the exercise by sitting in a circle, in a large well lit and well ventilated room.

Equipment required: a flip-chart pad, white or blackboard and marking pen or chalk.

Time required: 45 minutes to 1 hour.

The activity:
Group members remain in a circle and a volunteer from the group is invited to facilitate a group discussion for about 30 minutes. The facilitator conducts the discussion using a directive style of facilitation. That is to say that she uses the following sorts of facilitative interventions:

1. direct questions;
2. summaries of what has been said;
3. interventions which encourage each person in the group to speak;
4. interventions which 'shut out' the overeager speaker, and so on.

At the end of the discussion the volunteer facilitator sums up what has been discussed.

At the end of the 30 minutes, a group discussion is held about the appropriateness or otherwise of the person's facilitation skills. Comments may be recorded on a flip-chart sheet or on the white or black board. A discussion is also held on the relative value of this style of interventions when compared to other styles described in this series of activities.

Evaluation procedure:
At the end of the activity each member, in turn, is asked to say two things that they learned from the activity. They are then invited to say (a) what they liked least about it, and (b) what they liked most about it. Alternatively, participants may be invited to write down their thoughts about the activity, for their own use.

Activity number thirty

Aim of the activity: to explore a non-directive style of group facilitation.

Number of participants recommended: between 5 and 25.

Environmental considerations: participants should start the exercise by sitting in a circle, in a large well lit and well ventilated room.

Equipment required: a flip-chart pad, white or blackboard and marking pen or chalk.

Time required: 45 minutes to 1 hour.

The activity:
Group members remain in a circle and a volunteer from the group is invited to facilitate a group discussion for about 30 minutes. The facilitator uses a non-directive style of group facilitation. She restricts herself to those interventions that encourage the development of discussion, such as:

1. open-ended questions;
2. reflections;
3. empathy building statements.

She makes no attempt to lead or direct the discussion in any way and makes no attempt to sum up what has been talked about at the end of the 30 minutes.

At the end of the 30 minutes, a group discussion is held about the appropriateness or otherwise of the person's facilitation skills. Comments may be recorded on a flip-chart sheet or on the white or blackboard. A discussion is also held on the relative value of this style of interventions when compared to other styles described in this series of activities.

Evaluation procedure:
At the end of the activity each member, in turn, is asked to say two things that they learned from the activity. They are then invited to say (a) what they liked least about it, and (b) what they liked most about it. Alternatively, participants may be invited to write down their thoughts about the activity, for their own use.

Activity number thirty-one

Aim of the activity: to explore an interpretative style of group facilitation.

Number of participants recommended: between 5 and 25.

155

Environmental considerations: participants should start the exercise by sitting in a circle, in a large well lit and well ventilated room.

Equipment required: a flip-chart pad, white or blackboard and marking pen or chalk.

Time required: 45 minutes to 1 hour.

The activity:
Group members remain in a circle and a volunteer from the group is invited to facilitate a group discussion for about 30 minutes. The volunteer facilitator uses an interpretative style of group leadership. Thus she may offer comments on what is happening within the group (the group process) or she may offer interpretations of what people are saying in the group (the group content). Interpretative frameworks used in this exercise will depend upon the group members' experience, education and belief system. She may, for example, offer interpretations from one or more of the following interpretative frameworks:

1. psychodynamic;
2. behavioural;
3. symbolic interactionist;
4. religious;
5. sociological;
6. transactional analytical and so forth.

At the end of the 30 minutes, a group discussion is held about the appropriateness or otherwise of the person's facilitation skills. Comments may be recorded on a flip-chart sheet or on the white or black board. A discussion is also held on the relative value of this style of interventions when compared to other styles described in this series of activities.

Evaluation procedure:
At the end of the activity each member, in turn, is asked to say two things that they learned from the activity. They are then invited to say (a) what they liked least about it, and (b) what they liked most about it. Alternatively, participants may be invited to write down their thoughts about the activity, for their own use.

Activity number thirty-two

Aim of the activity: to explore a non-interpretative style of group facilitation.

Number of participants recommended: between 5 and 25.

Environmental considerations: participants should start the exercise by sitting in a circle, in a large well lit and well ventilated room.

Equipment required: a flip-chart pad, white or blackboard and marking pen or chalk.

Time required: 45 minutes to 1 hour.

The activity:
Group members remain in a circle and a volunteer from the group is invited to facilitate a group discussion for about 30 minutes. During the discussion, the facilitator encourages group members to offer interpretations of either what is happening within the group (the group process) or interpretations of what is being said in the group (the group content). She makes no interpretations herself of either what is going on nor what is being said.

At the end of the 30 minutes, a group discussion is held about the appropriateness or otherwise of the person's facilitation skills. Comments may be recorded on a flip-chart sheet or on the white or blackboard. A discussion is also held on the relative value of this style of interventions when compared to other styles described in this series of activities.

Evaluation procedure:
At the end of the activity each member, in turn, is asked to say two things that they learned from the activity. They are then invited to say (a) what they liked least about it, and (b) what they liked most about it. Alternatively, participants may be invited to write down their thoughts about the activity, for their own use.

Activity number thirty-three

Aim of the activity: to explore a structured style of group facilitation.

157

Number of participants recommended: between 5 and 25.

Environmental considerations: participants should start the exercise by sitting in a circle, in a large well lit and well ventilated room.

Equipment required: a flip-chart pad, white or blackboard and marking pen or chalk.

Time required: 45 minutes to 1 hour.

The activity:
Group members remain in a circle and a volunteer from the group is invited to facilitate a group discussion for about 30 minutes. The facilitator offers the group a structured activity to carry out, that will take about 20 minutes to complete. Examples of such activities can be gleaned from the many titles that appear in the bibliography appending this book. The final ten minutes of the period is allowed for a free discussion of what happened during the structured activity.

At the end of the 30 minutes, a group discussion is held about the appropriateness or otherwise of the person's facilitation skills. Comments may be recorded on a flip-chart sheet or on the white or blackboard. A discussion is also held on the relative value of this style of interventions when compared to other styles described in this series of activities.

Evaluation procedure:
At the end of the activity each member, in turn, is asked to say two things that they learned from the activity. They are then invited to say (a) what they liked least about it, and (b) what they liked most about it. Alternatively, participants may be invited to write down their thoughts about the activity, for their own use.

Activity number thirty-four

Aim of the activity: to explore an unstructuring style of group facilitation.

Number of participants recommended: between 5 and 25.

Environmental considerations: participants should start the exercise by sitting in a circle, in a large well lit and well ventilated room.

Equipment required: a flip-chart pad, white or blackboard and marking pen or chalk.

Time required: 45 minutes to 1 hour.

The activity:
Group members remain in a circle and a volunteer from the group is invited to facilitate a group discussion for about 30 minutes. The facilitator suggests that the group decides how it would like to use the thirty minutes and makes no attempt to structure the time in any way at all. She does not attempt to draw up an agenda with the group, nor suggest a plan of action derived from what individual members suggests. She merely allows the group discussion to unfold and makes no attempt to structure it in any way. She may, of course, join in with the discussion but in no sense acts as a chairperson. Instead, she encourages the group to find its own way.

At the end of the 30 minutes, a group discussion is held about the appropriateness or otherwise of the person's facilitation skills. Comments may be recorded on a flip-chart sheet or on the white or blackboard. A discussion is also held on the relative value of this style of interventions when compared to other styles described in this series of activities.

Evaluation procedure:
At the end of the activity each member, in turn, is asked to say two things that they learned from the activity. They are then invited to say (a) what they liked least about it, and (b) what they liked most about it. Alternatively, participants may be invited to write down their thoughts about the activity, for their own use.

Activity number thirty-five

Aim of the activity: to explore a cathartic style of group facilitation.

Number of participants recommended: between 5 and 25.

Environmental considerations: participants should start the exercise by sitting in a circle, in a large well lit and well ventilated room.

Equipment required: a flip-chart pad, white or blackboard and marking pen or chalk.

159

Time required: 45 minutes to 1 hour.

The activity:
This is an activity for a group that has had some training in handling the emotional release of others. Group members remain in a circle and a volunteer from the group is invited to facilitate a group discussion for about 30 minutes.

The facilitator invokes a discussion around the topic of how people in the group are feeling. During the discussion, she invites anyone who is emotionally stirred by the discussion to allow themselves to express their feelings and to note any insights that such release may bring. A wide range of cathartic interventions may be used. For examples of such interventions, see Heron (1977) and Burnard (1985).

At the end of the 30 minutes, a group discussion is held about the appropriateness or otherwise of the person's facilitation skills. Comments may be recorded on a flip-chart sheet or on the white or blackboard. A discussion is also held on the relative value of this style of interventions when compared to other styles described in this series of activities.

Evaluation procedure:
At the end of the activity each member, in turn, is asked to say two things that they learned from the activity. They are then invited to say (a) what they liked least about it, and (b) what they liked most about it. Alternatively, participants may be invited to write down their thoughts about the activity, for their own use.

Activity number thirty-six

Aim of the activity: to explore a non-cathartic style of group facilitation.

Number of participants recommended: between 5 and 25.

Environmental considerations: participants should start the exercise by sitting in a circle, in a large well lit and well ventilated room.

Equipment required: a flip-chart pad, white or blackboard and marking pen or chalk.

Time required: 45 minutes to 1 hour.

The activity:
Group members remain in a circle and a volunteer from the group is invited to facilitate a group discussion for about 30 minutes. The facilitator invokes a discussion on an emotive issue but does not encourage the free expression of emotion. Instead, she practises 'lightening' the atmosphere by the use of such interventions as:

1. the use of humour;
2. a change of topic;
3. switching the discussion to another member of the group and so on.

At the end of the 30 minutes, a group discussion is held about the appropriateness or otherwise of the person's facilitation skills. Comments may be recorded on a flip-chart sheet or on the white or blackboard. A discussion is also held on the relative value of this style of interventions when compared to other styles described in this series of activities.

Evaluation procedure:
At the end of the activity each member, in turn, is asked to say two things that they learned from the activity. They are then invited to say (a) what they liked least about it, and (b) what they liked most about it. Alternatively, participants may be invited to write down their thoughts about the activity, for their own use.

Activity number thirty-seven

Aim of the activity: to explore a disclosing style of group facilitation.

Number of participants recommended: between 5 and 25.

Environmental considerations: participants should start the exercise by sitting in a circle, in a large well lit and well ventilated room.

Equipment required: a flip-chart pad, white or blackboard and marking pen or chalk.

Time required: 45 minutes to 1 hour.

The activity:
Group members remain in a circle and a volunteer from the group is invited to facilitate a group discussion for about 30 minutes. The facilitator invites the group to join in a discussion on any topic and during that discussion, the facilitator offers her own points of view as an equal member of the group. She also allows herself to share something of how she is feeling with the group and thus 'personalizes' the discussion.

At the end of the 30 minutes, a group discussion is held about the appropriateness or otherwise of the person's facilitation skills. Comments may be recorded on a flip-chart sheet or on the white or blackboard. A discussion is also held on the relative value of this style of interventions when compared to other styles described in this series of activities.

Evaluation procedure:
At the end of the activity each member, in turn, is asked to say two things that they learned from the activity. They are then invited to say (a) what they liked least about it, and (b) what they liked most about it. Alternatively, participants may be invited to write down their thoughts about the activity, for their own use.

Activity number thirty-eight

Aim of the activity: to explore a non-disclosing style of group facilitation.

Number of participants recommended: between 5 and 25.

Environmental considerations: participants should start the exercise by sitting in a circle, in a large well lit and well ventilated room.

Equipment required: a flip-chart pad, white or blackboard and marking pen or chalk.

Time required: 45 minutes to 1 hour.

The activity:
Group members remain in a circle and a volunteer from the group is invited to facilitate a group discussion for about 30 minutes. The facilitator invites the group to join in a discussion on any topic and

during that discussion, the facilitator does not offer her own points of view on the topic under discussion. Neither does she share with the group how she is feeling. In this sense, she remains a 'blank' to the group.

It is arguable that if this exercise is being carried out as the first exercise that a particular group takes part in, then any observations that group members make about the facilitator will necessarily be 'projections' on the part of that group member. In other words, as the group member knows nothing about the group facilitator (because she is remaining 'non-disclosing'), then anything that another person says about her is likely to be actually true of that person, himself!

At the end of the 30 minutes, a group discussion is held about the appropriateness or otherwise of the person's facilitation skills. Comments may be recorded on a flip-chart sheet or on the white or blackboard. A discussion is also held on the relative value of this style of interventions when compared to other styles described in this series of activities.

Evaluation procedure:
At the end of the activity each member, in turn, is asked to say two things that they learned from the activity. They are then invited to say (a) what they liked least about it, and (b) what they liked most about it. Alternatively, participants may be invited to write down their thoughts about the activity, for their own use.

References

Alberti, R.E. and Emmons, M.L. (1982) *Your Perfect Right: A Guide to Assertive Living*, Impact, San Luis Obispo, California.

Argyle, M. (1975) *The Psychology of Interpersonal Behaviour*, Penguin, Harmondsworth.

Atwood, A.H. (1979) The mentor in clinical practice. *Nursing Outlook*, **27**, 714–717.

Bandler, R. and Grinder, J. (1975) *The Structure of Magic: Volume I. A Book About Language and Therapy*, Science and Behaviour Books, California.

Bateson, C.D. and Coke, J.S. (1981) Empathy: a source of altruistic motivation for helping? In *Altruism and Helping Behaviour: Social, Personality and Developmental Perspectives* J.P. Rushton and R.M. Sorventino, Lawrence Erlbaum Associates, New Jersey.

Blake, R. and Mouton, J. (1976) The D/D matrix: scientific methods. Cited in *Six Category Intervention Analysis* (J. Heron), 1975, Human Potential Research Project, University of Surrey, Guildford.

Blaney, J. (1974) Program development and curricular authority. In *Program Development in Education* eds J. Blaney, I. Housego and G. McIntoxh, University of British Colombia, Vancouver.

Boydel, T. (1976) *Experimental Learning*, Manchester Monography No 5, Department of Adult and Higher Education, University of Manchester, Manchester.

Bond, M. (1986) *Stress and Self-Awareness: A Guide for Nurses*, Heinemann, London.

Bond, M. and Kilty, J. (1986) *Practical Methods of Dealing With Stress* , 2nd Edn, Human Potential Research Project, University of Surrey, Guildford.

Brandes, D. and Phillips, R. (1984) *The Gamester's Handbook*, Vol. 2, Hutchinson, London.

Brookfield, S.D. (1986) *Understanding and Facilitating Adult Learning: A Comprehensive Analysis of Principles and Effective Practices*, Open University Press, Milton Keynes.

Brookfield, S.D. (1987) *Developing Critical Thinkers: Challenging Adults to Explore Alternative Ways of Thinking and Acting*, Open University Press, Milton Keynes.

Buber, M. (1958) *I and Thou*, 2nd Edn, Scribner, New York.

Buber, M. (1966) *The Knowledge of Man: a philosophy of the interhuman*, (ed. M. Friedman, trans. R.G. Smith), Harper and Row, New York.

Bullock, A. and Stallybrass, O. (1977) *The Fontana Dictionary of Modern Thought*, Fontana/Collins, London.

Burnard, P. (1985) *Learning Human Skills: A Guide for Nurses*, Heinemann, London.

Burnard, P. (1987a) *A Study of the Ways in Which Experiential Learning Methods Are Used to Develop Interpersonal Skills in Nurses in Canada and the United States*, National Florence Nightingale Memorial Committee, London.

Burnard, P. (1987b) Self and peer assessment. *Senior Nurse*, **6**, (5), 16–17.

Burnard, P. (1989) *Counselling Skills for Health Professionals*, Chapman and Hall, London.

Burnard, P. and Morrison, P. (1988) Nurses perceptions of their inter-personal skills: a descriptive study using Six Category Intervention Analysis. *Nurse Education Today*, **8**, 266–72.

Burton, A. (1975) The mentoring dynamic in the therapeutic transformation. *Amer. J. Psychoanalysis*, **37**, 115–22.

Callner, D. and Ross, S. (1978) The assessment and training of asser-tiveness skills with drug addicts: a preliminary study. *Intern. J. Addic-tions*, **13**, (2), 227–30.

Campbell, A. (1984) *Paid to Care?*, SPCK, London.

Collins, G.C. and Scott, P. (1979) Everybody who makes it has a mentor. *Harvard Business Review*, **56**, 89–101.

Darling, L.A.W. (1984) What do nurses want in a mentor? *J. Nursing Admin.*, October, 42–4.

Dewey, J. (1916) *Democracy and Education*, published in 1966 by Free Press, London.

Dewey, J. (1938) *Experience and Education*, published in 1971 by Collier Macmillan, London.

Edelstein, B. and Eisler, R. (1976) Effects of modelling and modelling with instruction and feedback on the behavioural components of social skills. *Behaviour Therapy*, **4**, 382–9.

Ellis, R. and Whittington, D. (1981) *A Guide to Social Skill Training*, Croom Helm, London.

Egan, G. (1986) *The Skilled Helper*, 3rd Edn, Brooks/Cole, Monterey.

Falloon, I., Lindley, P., McDonald, R. and Marks, I. (1977) Social skills training of out patient groups. *Brit. J. Psychiatry*, 131, 599–609.

Fay, A. (1978) *Making Things Better by Making Them Worse*, Hawthorne, New York.

FEU (1983) *Curriculum Opportunity: A Map of Experiential Learning in Entry Requirements to Higher and Further Education Award Bearing Courses*, Further Education Unit, London.

Fielding, R.G. and Llewelyn, S.P. (1987) Communication training in nurs-ing may damage your health and enthusiasm: some warnings. *J. Advan. Nursing*, **12**, 281–90.

Frankl, V.E. (1975) *The Unconscious God*, Simon and Schuster, New York.

Freire, P. (1972) *Pedagogy of the Oppressed*, Penguin, Harmondsworth.

Gendlin, E.T. and Beebe, J. (1968) An experiential approach to group therapy. *J. Res. Develop. Education*, **1**, 19–29.

Gross, R. (1977) *The Lifelong Learner*, Simon and Schuster, New York.

Grossman, R. (1985) Some reflections on Abraham Maslow, *J. Human. Psych.*, **25**, (4), 31–4.

Hall, C. (1954) *A Primer of Freudian Psychology*, Mentor Books, New York.

Halmos, P. (1965) *The Faith of the Counsellors*, Constable, London.

Hampden-Turner, C. (1966) An existential learning theory, *J. Appl. Behav. Sc.*, **12**, 4.

Hanks, L., Belliston, L. and Edwards, D. (1977) *Design Yourself*, Kauf-man, Los Altos, California.

Hargie, O., Saunders, C. and Dickson, D. (1981) *Social Skills in Interpersonal Communication*, 2nd Edn, Croom Helm, London.

Heidegger, M. (1927) *Being and Time*, published in 1962, Harper and Row, New York.

Heron, J. (1970) *The Phenomenology of the Gaze*, Human Potential Research Project, University of Surrey, Guildford.

Heron, J. (1973) *Experiential Training Techniques*, Human Potential Research Project, University of Surrey, Guildford.

Heron, J. (1975) *Behaviour Analysis in Education and Training*, Human Potential Research Project, University of Surrey, Guildford.

Heron, J. (1977) *Catharsis in Human Development*, Human Potential Research Project, University of Surrey, Guildford.

Heron, J. (1981) Philosophical basis for a new paradigm. In P. Reason and J. Rowan *Human Inquiry: A Sourcebook of New Paradigm Research* (eds P. Reason and J. Rowan), Wiley, Chichester.

Heron, J. (1982) *Education of the Affect*, Human Potential Research Project, University of Surrey, Guildford.

Heron, J. (1986) *Six Category Intervention Analysis*, 2nd Edn, Human Potential Research Project, University of Surrey, Guildford.

Hewitt, J. (1977) *Meditation*, Hodder and Stoughton, Sevenoaks, Kent.

Husserl, E. (1931) *Ideas: General Introduction to Pure Phenomenology*, (trans by G. Boyce), Allen and Unwin, London.

Jarvis, P. (1983) *Professional Education*, Croom Helm, London.

Jenkins, E. (1987) *Facilitating Self-Awareness: a Learning Package Combining Group Work with Computer Assisted Learning*, Open Software Library, Wigan.

Johns, G. and Morris, N. (1988) Nursing hopes. *Open Mind*, **30**, 16–17.

Jourard, S. (1964) *The Transparent Self*, Van Nostrand, Princeton, New Jersey.

Jourard, S. (1971) *Self-Disclosure: an Experimental Analysis of the Transparent Self*, Wiley, New York.

Kalisch, B.J. (1971) Strategies for developing nurse empathy. *Nursing Outlook*, **19**, (11), 714–17.

Keeton, M. *et al.* (1976) *Experiential Learning*, Jossey Bass, San Francisco, California.

Kelly, G.A. (1970) A brief introduction to personal construct theory. In *Perspectives in Construct Theory* (ed. D. Bannister), Academic Press, New York.

Kelly, G.A. (1969) The autobiography of a theory. In *Clinical Psychology and Personality: The Selected Papers of George Kelly* (B. Maher), Wiley, pp. 97–103.

Kilty, J. (1976) *Self and Peer Assessment*, Human Potential Research Project, University of Surrey, Guildford.

Kilty, J. (1983) *Experiential Learning*, Human Potential Research Project, University of Surrey, Guildford.

Kilty, J. (1987) *Staff Development for Nurse Education: Practioners Supporting Students: A Report of a 5-Day Development Workshop*, Human Potential Research Project, University of Surrey, Guildford.

King, E.C. (1984) *Affective Education in Nursing: A guide to teaching and assessment*, Aspen, Maryland.

Knowles, M.S. (1975) *Self Directed Learning*, Cambridge Books, New York.

Knowles, M.S. (1978) *The Adult Leaner: A Neglected Species*, 2nd Edn, Gulf, Texas.

Knowles, M.S. (1980) *The Modern Practice of Adult Education: From Pedagogy to Andragogy*, 2nd Edn, Follett, Chicago.

Knowles, M.S. and Associates, (1984) *Andragogy in Action: Applying Modern Principles of Adult Learning*, Jossey Bass, San Francisco, California.

Kirschenbaum, H. (1979) *On Becoming Carl Rogers*, Dell, New York.

Koberg, D. and Bagnal, J. (1981) *The Revised All New Universal Traveler: A Soft-Systems Guide to Creativity, Problem-Solving and the Process of Reaching Goals*, Kaufmann, Los Altos, California.

Kolb, D. (1984) *Experiential Learning*, Prentice Hall, Englewood Cliffs, New Jersey.

Lawton, D. (1973) *Social Change, Educational Therapy and Curriculum Planning*, Hodder and Stoughton, London.

Luft, J. (1969) *Of Human Interaction: The Johari Model*, Mayfield, Palo Alto, California.

Macquarrie, J. (1973) *Existentialism*, Penguin, Harmondsworth.

Maslow, A. (1972) *Motivation and Personality*, 2nd Edn, Harper and Row, New York.

Mayeroff, M. (1972) *On Caring*, Harper and Row, New York.

Michelson, L., Sugari, D., Wood, R. and Kazadin, A. (1983) *Social Skills Assessment and Training with Children*, Plenum Press, New York.

Mocker, D.W. and Spear, G.E. (1982) *Lifelong Learning: Formal, Non-formal and Self-Directed*, The ERIC Clearinghouse on Adult Career and Vocational Education, Columbus, Ohio.

Moreno, J.L. (1959) *Psychodrama*, Vol. II, Beacon House Press, Beacon House, New York.

Moreno, J.L. (1969) *Psychodrama*, Vol. III, Beacon House Press, Beacon House, New York.

Moreno, J.L. (1977) *Psychodrama*, Vol. I, 4th Edn, Beacon House Press, Beacon House, New York.

Morris, D. (1977) *Manwatching: a field guide to human behaviour*, Triad/Panther, London.

Murgatroyd, S. (1986) *Counselling and Helping*, Methuen, London.

Naranjo, C. and Ornstein, R.E. (1971) *On the Psychology of Meditation*, Allen and Unwin, London.

Nelson-Jones, R. (1981) *The Theory and Practice of Counselling Psychology*, Holt, Rinehart and Winston, London.

Newble, D. and Cannon, R. (1987) *A Handbook for Medical Teachers*, 2nd Edn, MTP Press, Lancaster.

Open University Coping With Crisis Group (1987) *Running Workshops: A Guide for Trainers in the Helping Professions*, Croom Helm, London.

Ouspensky, P.D. (1988) *Conscience: The Search for Truth*, Arkana, London.

Patton, M.Q. (1982) *Practical Evaluation*, Sage, Beverly Hills, California.

Peters, R.S. (1966) *Ethics and Education*, Allen and Unwin, London.

Peters, R.S. (1972) Education as Initiation. In *Philosophical Analysis and*

Education (ed. R.D. Archambault), Routledge and Kegan Paul, London.

Pfeiffer, J.W. and Goodstein, L.D. (1982) *The 1982 Annual for Facilitators, Trainers and Consultants*, University Associates, San Diego, California.

Pirsig, R. (1974) *The Zen of Motor Cycle Maintenance*, Arrow, London.

Polyani, M. (1958) *Personal Knowledge*, University of Chicago Press, Chicago.

Postman, N. and Weingartner, C.W. (1969) *Teaching as a Subversive Activity*, Penguin, Harmondsworth.

Pring, R. (1976) *Knowledge and Schooling*, Open Books, London.

Riebel, L. (1984) A homeopathic model of psychotherapy, *J. Humanistic Psych.*, **24**, (1) 9–48.

Rogers, C.R. (1951) *Client-Centred Therapy*, Constable, London.

Rogers, C.R. (1967) *On Becoming a Person*, Constable, London.

Rogers, C.R. (1983) *Freedom to Learn for the Eighties*, Merrill, Columbus.

Rogers, C.R. (1985) Toward a more human science of the person. *J. Human. Psych.*, **25**, (4), 7–24.

Rogers, C.R. and Stevens, B. (1967) *Person to Person: The Problem of Being Human*, Real People Press, Lafayette, California.

Ryle, G. (1949) *The Concept of Mind*, Peregrine, Harmondsworth.

Sartre, J-P. (1956) *Being and Nothingness*, Philosophical Library, New York.

Schulman, E.D. (1982) *Intervention in Human Services: a Guide to Skills and Knowledge*, 3rd Edn, C.V. Mosby, St Louis, Missouri.

Scriven, M. (1967) The Methodology of Evaluation. In *Perspectives in Curriculum Evaluation* ed. R.W. Tyler), Rand McNally, Chicago.

Searle, J.R. (1983) *Intentionality: An Essay in Philosophy of the Mind*, Cambridge University Press, Cambridge.

Trower, P. (ed.) (1984) *Radical Approaches to Social Skills Training*, Croom Helm, London.

Vonnegut, K. (1967) *Mother Night*, Cape, London.

Whitehead, A.N. (1932) *The Aims of Education*, Benn, London.

Whorf, B.J. (1956) *Language, Thought and Reality: Selected Writings*, Technology Press of Massachusetts Institute of Technology, Cambridge, Mass.

Recommended and Further Reading

CHAPTER ONE: EXPERIENTIAL LEARNING

Archambault, R.D. (ed.) (1964) *John Dewey on Education: Selected Writings*, Random House, New York.

Boot, R. and Reynolds, M. (1983) *Learning and Experience in Formal Education*, Manchester Monograph, Department of Adult and Higher Education, University of Manchester.

Boud, D. (ed.) (1973) *Experiential Learning Techniques in Higher Education*, Human Potential Research Project, University of Surrey, Guildford, Surrey.

Boud, D. and Prosser, M.T. (1980) Sharing responsibility: staff–student cooperation in learning. *Brit. J. Educ. Tech.*, **11**, (1), 24–35.

Bower, G.H. and Hilgard, E.R. (1981) *Theories of Learning* (5th Edn), Prentice Hall, Englewood Cliffs, New Jersey.

Bridges, W. (1973) The three faces of humanistic education. In *Curriculum Development: Issues and Insights* (eds D.E. Orlosky and B.O. Smith), Rand McNally, Chicago.

Brocket, R. and Hiemstra, R. (1985) Bridging the theory–practice gap in self-directed learning. In *Self-Directed Learning: From Theory to Practice. New Directions for Continuing Education No 25* (ed. S.D. Brookfield), Jossey Bass, San Francisco, Cal.

Brown, G. (1971) *Human Teaching for Human Learning*, Viking Press, New York.

Brown, I.B. (ed.) (1975) *The Living Classroom*, Esalen/Viking, Cal.

Chene, A. (1983) The concept of autonomy in adult education: a philosophical discussion. *Adult Education Quarterly*, **32**, (1), 38–47.

Coleman, J.S. (1982) Experiential learning and information assimilation: towards an appropriate mix. *Child and Youth Services*, **14**, 3–4, 12–20.

Conrad, D. and Hedin, D. (1982) The impact of experiential education on adolescent development. *Child and Youth Services*, **4**, 3–4, 57–76.

Cunningham, P.M. (1983) Helping students extract meaning from experience. In *Helping Adults Learn How to Learn: New Directions for Continuing Education No 19* (ed. R.M. Smith), Jossey Bass, San Francisco, Cal.

Davis, C.M. (1981) Affective education for the health professions. *Physical Therapy*, **61**, (11), 1587–93.

Dowd, C. (1983) Learning through experience. *Nursing Times*, 27th July, 50–2.

Du Bois, E.E. (1982) Human resource development: expanding role. In *Materials and Methods in Adult and Continuing Education* (ed. C. Klevens), Klevins Publications, Canoga Park, Cal.

Famighetti, R.A. (1981) Experiential learning: the close encounters of the institutional kind. *Gerontology and Geriatric Education*, **2**, (2), 129–32.

Fox, F.E. (1983) The spiritual core of experiential education. *J. Experiential Education*, **16**, (1), 3–6.

Freire, P. (1985) *The Politics of Education*, Bergin and Garvey, South Hadley, Mass.

Gager, R. (1982) Experiential education: strengthening the learning process. *Child and Youth Services*, 4, (3–4), 31–9.

Guba, E.G. (1978) *Towards a Methodology of Naturalistic Inquiry in Educational Evaluation*, SE Monograph Series in Evaluation No 8, Center for the Study of Evaluation, University of California., Los Angeles, Cal.

Hamrick, M. and Stone, C. (1979) Promoting experiential learning. *Health Education*, **10**, (4), 38–41.

Hendricks, G. and Fadiman, J. (eds) (1976) *Transpersonal Education: a Curriculum for Feeling and Being*, Prentice Hall, Englewood Cliffs, New Jersey.

Heron, J. (1981) *Experiential Research: a New Paradigm*, Human Potential Research Project, University of Surrey, Guildford, Surrey.

Hudson, A. (1983) The politics of experiential learning. In *Learning and Experience in Formal Education* (eds R. Boot and M. Reynolds), Manchester Monograph, Department of Adult and Higher Education, University of Manchester.

Hunter, E. (1972) *Encounter in the Classroom*, Holt Rinehart and Winston, New York.

Jarvis, P. (1987) *Adult Learning in the Social Context*, Croom Helm, London.

Levison, R.H. (1979) Experiential education abroad. *Teaching Sociology*, **6**, (4), 415–19.

Lewin, K. (1969) Quasi-stationary social equilibria and the problems of permanent change. In *The Planning of Change* (eds W.G. Bennis, K.D. Benn and R. Chin), Holt Rheinhart and Winston, New York.

Lipsett, L. and Avakian, N.A. (1981) Assessing experiential learning. *Lifelong Learning: The Adult Years*, **5**, (2), 18–22.

Lomas, P. (1973) *True and False Experience*, Allen Lane, London.

Menson, B. (ed.) (1982) *Building on Experiences in Adult Development: New Directions for Experiential Learning No 16*, Jossey Bass, San Francisco, Cal.

Mouton, J.S. and Blake, R.R. (1984) *Synergogy: A New Strategy for Education Training and Development*, Jossey Bass, San Francisco, Cal.

Noble, P. (1983) *Formation of Freirian Facilitators*, Latino Institute, Chicago.

Nyberg, D. (ed.) (1975) *The Philosophy of Open Education*, Routledge and Kegan Paul, London.

Ringuette, E.L. (1983) A note on experiential learning in professional training. *J. Clinical Psychology*, **39**, (2), 302–4.

Rogers, C.R. (1972) The facilitation of significant learning. In *The Psychology of Open Learning and Teaching: an inquiry approach* (eds L. Silberman, J.S. Allender and J.M. Yanoff), Little Brown and Co, Boston, Mass.

Schafer, B.P. and Morgan, M.K. (1980) An experiential learning laboratory: a new dimension in teaching mental health skills. *Issues in Mental Health Nursing*, **2**, (3), 47–57.

Shaffer, J.B.P. (1978) *Humanistic Psychology*, Prentice Hall, Englewood Cliffs, New Jersey.

Shropshire, C.O. (1981) Group experiential learning in adult education. *J. Contin. Educ. Nursing*, **12**, (6), 5–9.

Soth, N. (1981) Experiential education from a cultural viewpoint: the peer evaluation meeting as a ritual of enculturation. *Alternative Higher Education*, **16**, (2), 88–95.

Stitch, T.F. (1983) Experiential therapy. *J. Exper. Educ.*, **5**, (3), 23–30.

Tough, A.M. (1982) *International Changes: A Fresh Approach to Helping People Change*, Cambridge Books, New York.

CHAPTER TWO: EXPERIENTIAL LEARNING METHODS

Barker, D. (1980) *T.A. and Training*, Gower, Aldershot, UK.

Canfield, J. and Wells, H.C. (1976) *100 Ways to Enhance Self-Concept in the Classroom*, Prentice Hall, Englewood Cliffs, New Jersey.

Carkhuff, R.R. (1969) *Helping and Human Relations: A Primer for Lay Professional Helpers Volume One: Selection and Training*, Holt Reinhart and Winston, New York.

Dahl, J. (1984) Structured experience: a risk-free approach to reality-based learning. *J. Nursing Educ.*, **23**, (1), 34–7.

Di Fabio, S. and Ackerhalt, J.E. (1978) Teaching the use of restraint through role-play. *Perspec. Psych. Care*, **15**, (5/6), 218–22.

Egan, G. (1976) *Interpersonal Living*, Brooks/Cole, Monterey, Cal.

Ernst, S. and Goodison, L. (1981) *In Our Own Hands: A Book of Self-Help Therapy*, The Women's Press, London.

Eskin, F. (1982) Learning team skills: an experience based model. *J. Management Develop.*, **1**, (1), 3–9.

Ferruci, P. (1982) *What We May Be*, Turnstone Press, Wellingborough.

Francis, D. and Woodcock, M. (1982) *Fifty Activities for Self-Development*, Gower, Aldershot.

Heron, J. (1977) *Six Category Intervention Analysis: Interpersonal Skills Course*, Human Potential Research Project, University of Surrey, Guildford.

James, M. and Jongeward, D. (1971) *Born to Win*, Addison-Wesley, Reading, Mass.

Johnson, D.W. and Johnson, F.P. (1975) *Joining Together: Group Therapy and Group Skills*, Prentice Hall, Englewood Cliffs, New Jersey.

Joynt, P. and Rylter, M.L. (1982) Experimenting with experience. *J. Europ. Indust. Training*, **5**, (7), 23–6.

McCabe, O.L. (1977) *Changing Human Behaviour: Current Therapies and Future Directions*, Grune and Stratton, New York.

Rogers, C.R. (1970) *On Encounter Groups*, Penguin, Harmondsworth.

Schutz, W.C. (1982) *Elements of Encounter*, Irvington, New York.

Van Ments, M. (1983) *The Effective Use of Role-Play*, Kogan Page, London.

CHAPTER THREE: INTERPERSONAL SKILLS

Counselling

Axelson, J.A. (1985) *Counseling and Development in a Multicultural Society*, Brooks/Cole, Monterey, Cal.

Baruth, L.G. (1987) *An Introduction to the Counselling Profession*, Prentice Hall, Englewood Cliffs, New Jersey.

Belkin, G.S. (1984) *Introduction to Counseling*, Brown, Dubuque, Iowa.

Black, K. (1983) *Short-Term Counselling: A Humanistic Approach for the Helping Professions*, Addison-Wesley, London.

Blocher, D.H. (1987) *The Professional Counselor*, Macmillan, New York.

Bohart, A.C. and Todd, J. (1988) *Foundations of Clinical and Counselling Psychology*, Harper and Row, New York.

Bolger, A.W. (ed.) (1982) *Counselling in Britain: a Reader*, Batsford Academic, London.

Braswell, M. and Seay, T. (1984) *Approaches to Counselling and Psychotherapy*, Waverly, Prospect Heights, Ill.

Brown, D. and Srebalus, D.J. (1988) *An Introduction to the Counselling Process*, Prentice Hall, Englewood Cliffs, New Jersey.

Burnard, P. (1987) Counselling: basic principles in nursing. *The Professional Nurse*, **2**, (9), 278–80.

Burnard, P. (1987) Counselling skills. *J. District Nursing*, **6**, (7), 157–9.

Calnan, J. (1983) *Talking with Patients*, Heinemann, London.

Campbell, A.V. (ed.) (1987) *A Dictionary of Pastoral Care*, Crossroads, New York.

Carkuff, R.R. and Pierce, R.M. (1975) *Trainer's Guide: The Art of Helping*, Human Resources Development Press, Amerhurst, Mass.

Carkuff, R.R., Pierce, R.M. and Cannon, J.R. (1977) *The Art of Helping III*, Human Resources Development Press, Amerhurst, Mass.

Cavanagh, M.E. (1982) *The Counselling Experience: Understanding and Living It*, Brooks/Cole, Monterey, Cal.

Collins, M. (1983) *Communication in Health Care*, C.V. Mosby, St Louis, Miss.

Corey, F. (1982) *I Never Knew I Had a Choice* (2nd Edn), Brooks/Cole, Monterey, Cal.

Corey, G. (1977) *Theory and Practice of Counselling and Psychotherapy*, Brooks/Cole, Monterey, Cal.

Cormier, L.S. (1987) *The Professional Counselor: A Process Guide to Helping*, Prentice Hall, Englewood Cliffs, New Jersey.

Edwards, P.B. (1977) *Leisure Counselling Techniques: Individual and Group Counselling Step-by-Step* (Revised Edn), University Publishers, Los Angeles, Cal.

Egan, G. (1977) *You and Me*, Brooks/Cole, Monterey, Cal.

Egan, G. (1986) *Exercises in Helping Skills* (3rd Edn), Brooks/Cole, Monterey, Cal.

Gazda, G.M., Childers, D.K. and Brooks, D.K. (1987) *Foundations of Counselling and Human Services*, McGraw Hill, New York.

George, R.L. and Cristiani, T.S. (1986) *Counselling Theory and Practice*, Prentice Hall, Englewood Cliffs, New Jersey.

Gerber, S.K. (1986) *Responsive Therapy: A Systematic Approach to Counselling Skills*, Human Sciences Press, New York.

Gibson, R.L. and Mitchell, M.H. (1986) *Introduction to Counselling and Guidance*, Collier Macmillan, London.

Goodyear, R.K. and Sinnett, E.R. (1984) Current and Emerging Ethical Issues for Counseling Psychology. *Counseling Psychologist*, **12**, (3–4), 87–98.

Hackney, H. and Cormier, L.S. (1979) *Counselling Strategies and Objectives*, Prentice Hall, Englewood Cliffs, New Jersey.

Howard, G.S., Nance, D.W. and Meyers, P. (1987) *Adaptive Counselling and Therapy: A Systematic Approach to Selecting Effective Treatment*, Jossey Bass, San Francisco, Cal.

Janis, I.L. (ed.) (1982) *Counselling on Person Decisions: Theory and Research on Short-Term Helping Relationships*, Yale University Press, New Haven, Conn.

Johnson, S.E. (1987) *After a Child Dies: Counselling Bereaved Families*, Pringer, New York.

Kennedy, E. (1979) *On Becoming a Counsellor*, Gill and Macmillan, London.

Kottler, J.A. and Brown, R.W. (1985) *Introduction to Therapeutic Counselling*, Brooks/Cole, Monterey, Cal.

Lef'ebure, M. (ed.) (1985) *Conversation on Counselling Between a Doctor and a Priest: Dialogue and Trinity*, T & T Clark, Edinburgh.

Lewis, H. and Streitfield, H. (1971) *Growth Games*, Bantam Books, New York.

Maclean, D. and Gould, S. (1987) *The Helping Process: an Introduction*, Croom Helm, London.

Marriage Guidance Council (1983) *Aims, Beliefs and Organisation*, The National Marriage Guidance Council, Rugby, Warwickshire.

Morsund, J. (1985) *The Process of Counseling and Therapy*, Prentice Hall, Englewood Cliffs, New Jersey.

Mucchilelli, R. (1983) *Face-to-Face in the Counselling Relationship*, Macmillan, London.

Munro, E.A., Mantheir, R.J. and Small, J.J. (1979) *Counselling: a Skills Approach*, Methuen, Wellington, New Zealand.

Murgatroyd, S. and Woolfe, R. (1982) *Coping With Crisis: Understanding and Helping Persons in Need*, Harper and Row, London.

Nelson-Jones, R. (1983) *Practical Counselling Skills: A Psychological Skills Approach for the Helping Professions and for Voluntary Counsellors*, Holt Rinehart and Winston, London.

Nelson-Jones, R. (1984) *Personal Responsibility: Counselling and Therapy, an Integrative Approach*, Harper and Row, London.

Nelson-Jones, R. (1988) *Practical Counselling and Helping Skills: Helping Clients to Help Themselves*, Cassell, London.

Nicholson, J.A. and Golsan, G. (1983) *The Creative Counselor*, McGraw Hill, New York.

Noonan, E. (1983) *Counselling Young People*, Methuen, London.

Pederson, P. (ed.) (1987) *Handbook of Cross-Cultural Counselling and Therapy*, Praeger, London.

Procter, B. (1978) *Counselling Shop: An Introduction to the Theories and*

Techniques of Ten Approaches to Counselling, Deutsch, London.

Rogers, C.R. (1977) *On Personal Power*, Constable, London.

Rowan, J. (1983) *The Reality Game: A Guide to Humanistic Counselling and Psychotherapy*, Routledge and Kegan Paul, London.

Rubin, S.E. and Rubin, N.M. (ed.) (1988) *Contemporary Challenges to the Rehabilitation Counselling Profession*, Brookes, Baltimore.

Russell, M.L. (1986) *Behavioural Counselling in Medicine: Strategies for Modifying At-Risk Behaviour*, Oxford University Press, New York.

Shertzer, B. (1980) *Fundamentals of Counselling*, Houghton Mifflin, London.

Shilling, L.E. (1984) *Perspectives on Counselling Theories*, Prentice Hall, Englewood Cliffs, New Jersey.

Smith, V.M. and Bass, T.A. (1982) *Communication for the Health Care Team*, Harper and Row, London.

Stewart, W. (1979) *Health Service Counselling*, Pitman Medical, Tunbridge Wells, Kent.

Strongman, K.T. (1979) *Psychology for the Paramedical Professions*, Croom Helm, London.

Sue, D.W. (1981) *Counseling the Culturally Different*, Wiley, New York.

Talley, J.E. and Rockwell, W.J.K. (1985) *Counseling and Psychotherapy With College Students: A Guide to Treatment*, Praeger, New York.

Thompson, T.L. (1986) *Communication for Health Professionals*, Harper and Row, London.

Tipton, R.M. (1984) Trends and issues in the training and development of counselling psychologists. *Counselling Psychologist*, **12**, (3–4) 111–12.

Tschudin, V. (1986) *Counselling Skills for Nurses* (2nd Edn), Baillière Tindall, Eastbourne, East Sussex.

Tyler, M. (1978) *Advisory and Counselling Services for Young People*, HMSO, London.

Van Dogen, G. (1983) *Invisible Barriers: Pastoral Care and the Physically Disabled*, SPCK, London.

Walrond-Skinner, S. (1979) *Family and Marital Psychotherapy*, Routledge and Kegan Paul, London.

Webster, E.J. (1977) *Counseling with Parents of Handicapped Children*, Guidelines for Improving Communication, Grune and Stratton, New York.

Assertiveness

Alberti, R. (ed.) (1977) *Assertiveness: Innovations, Applications, Issues*, Impact, San Luis, Obispo, Cal.

Alberti, R. and Emmons, M. (1975) *Stand Up, Speak Out, Talk Back: The Key to Assertive Behaviour*, Impact, San Luis, Obispo, Cal.

Ausberger, D. (1979) *Anger and Assertiveness in Pastoral Care*, Fortress Press, Phil.

Baer, J. (1976) *How to Be Assertive (Not Aggressive): Women in Life, in Love and on the Job*, Signet, New York.

Bernard, J.M. (1980) Assertiveness in Children. *Psychological Reports*, **46**, 935–8.

Bower, S.A. and Bower, G.H. (1976) *Asserting Yourself*, Addison-Wesley, Reading, Mass.

Cianni-Surridge, M. and Horan, J. (1983) On wisdom of assertive job-seeking behaviour. *J. Counselling Psych.*, **30**, 209–14.

Clark, C. (1978) *Assertive Skills for Nurses*, Contemporary Publishing, Wakefield, Mass.

Dawley, H. and Wenrich, W. (1976) *Achieving Assertive Behaviour: a Guide to Assertive Training*, Brooks/Cole, Monterey, Cal.

Dickson, A. (1985) *A Woman in Your Own Right: Assertiveness and You*, Quartet Books, London.

Gordon, S. and Waldo, M. (1984) The effective of assertive training on couples' relationships. *Amer. J. Family Therapy*, **12**, 73–7.

Gormally, J. (1982) Evaluation of assertiveness: effects of gender, rater involvement and level of assertiveness. *Behaviour Therapy*, **13**, 219–25.

Hull, D. and Schroeder, H. (1979) Some interpersonal effects of assertion, non-assertion and aggression. *Behaviour Therapy*, **10**, 20–9.

Kelly, C. (1979) *Assertion Training: A Facilitator's Guide*, University Associates, La Jolla, Cal.

Lang, A.J. and Jakubowski, P. (1978) *The Assertive Option*, Research Press, Champagne.

Liberman, R.P., King, L.W., DeRisi, W.J. and McCann, M. (1976) *Personal Effectiveness*, Research Press, Champagne.

Meichenbaum, D. (1979) *Cognitive Behaviour Modification: an Integrative Approach*, Plenum Press, New York.

Moore, D. (1977) *Assertive Behaviour Training: An Annotated Bibliography*, Impact, San Luis, Obispo, Cal.

Osborn, S.M. and Harris, G.G. (1975) *Assertive Training for Women*, Charles C. Thomas, Springfield, Ill.

Palmer, M.E. and Deck, E.S. (1982) Assertiveness education: one method for teaching staff and patients. *Nurse Educator*, Winter, 36–9.

Phelps, S. and Austin, N. (1975) *The Assertive Woman*, Impact, San Luis Obispo, Cal.

Taubman, B. (1976) *How to Become an Assertive Woman*, Simon and Schuster, New York.

Zuker, E. (1983) *Mastering Assertiveness Skills*, American Management Association, New York.

Social skills

Argyle, M. (ed.) (1981) *Social Skills and Health*, Methuen, London.

Bandura, A. (1977) *Social Learning Theory*, Prentice Hall, Englewood Cliffs, New Jersey.

Bellack, A.S. and Hersen, M. (eds) (1979) *Research and Practice in Social Skills Training*, Plenum Press, New York.

Curran, J. and Monti, P. (eds) *Social Skills Training: A Practical Handbook for Assessment and Treatment*, Guildford, New York.

Duncan, S. and Fiske, D.W. (1977) *Face-to-Face Interaction: Research, Methods and Theory*, Lawrence Erlbaum Associates, Hillsdale, New Jersey.

Ellis, R. and Whittington, D. (eds) (1983) *New Directions in Social Skills Training*, Croom Helm, London.

French, P. (1983) *Social Skills for Nursing Practice*, Croom Helm, London.

Goffman, I. (1971) *The Presentation of Self in Everyday Life*, Penguin, Harmondsworth.

Harre, R. and Secord, P.F. (1972) *The Explanation of Social Behaviour*, Blackwell, Oxford.

L'Abate, L. and Milan, M. (eds) (1985) *Handbook of Social Skills Training and Research*, Wiley, New York.

McGuire, J. and Priestly, P. (1981) *Life After School: A Social Skills Curriculum*, Pergamon, Oxford.

Pope, B. (1986) *Social Skills Training for Psychiatric Nurses*, Harper and Row, London.

Priestley, P., McGuire, J., Flegg, D., Hemsley, V. and Welham, D. (1978) *Social Skills and Personal Problem Solving*, Tavistock, London.

Trower, P., Bryant, B.M. and Argyle, M. (eds) *Social Skills and Mental Health*, Methuen, London.

Trower, P., O'Mahony, J.M. and Dryden, W. (1982) Cognitive aspects of social failure: some implications for social skills training. *Brit. J. Guid. Counselling*, **10**, 176–84.

Wilkinson, J. and Canter, S. (1982) *Social Skills Training Manual: Assessment, Programme Design and Management of Training*, Wiley, Chichester.

Group facilitation

Bass, B.M. (1981) *Stogdill's Handbook of Leadership*, Free Press, New York.

Cartwright, D. and Zander, A. (1968) *Group Dynamics* (3rd Edn), Harper and Row, New York.

Cox, M. (1978) *Structuring the Therapeutic Process: Compromise With Chaos*, Pergamon, Oxford.

Fiedler, F.E. (1967) *A Theory of Effective Leadership*, McGraw Hill, New York.

Foulkes, S.M. (1964) *Therapeutic Group Analysis*, Allen and Unwin, London.

Garvin, C.D. (1981) *Contemporary Group Work*, Prentice Hall, Englewood Cliffs, New Jersey.

Hargie, O. (ed.) (1986) *A Handbook of Communication Skills*, Croom Helm, London.

Malamud, D.I. and Machover, S. (1955) *Towards Self-Understanding: Group Techniques in Self-Confrontation*, Charles C. Thomas, Springfield, Ill.

Philips, K. and Fraser, T. (1982) *The Management of Interpersonal Skills Training*, Gower, Aldershot.

Rogers, C.R. (1972) The facilitation of significant learning. In *The Psychology of Open Teaching and Learning* (eds M.L. Silberman, J.S. Allender and J.M. Yanoff), Little Brown and Co, Boston, Mass.

Satow, A. and Evans, M. (1983) *Working with Groups*, Tacade, Manchester.

Smith, P.B. (1980) *Group Processes and Personal Change*, Harper and Row, London.

Thomas, E.J. (1984) *Designing Interventions for the Helping Professions*, Sage, Beverly Hills, Cal.

CHAPTER FOUR: REMEMBERING AND SUPERVISING EXPERIENTIAL LEARNING

Bales, R.F. (1950) *Interaction Process Analysis: a method for the study of small groups*, Addison-Wesley, Cambridge, Mass.

Bolton, E.B. (1980) A conceptual analysis of the mentoring relationship in the career development of women. *Adult Education*, **30**, 195–207.

Boud, D., Keogh, R. and Walker, M. (1985) *Reflection: Turning Experience into Learning*, Kogan Page, London.

Brown, B.J. (1984) The Dean as mentor. *Nursing Health Care*, **5**, (2), 88–91.

Burnard, P. (1985) The teacher as facilitator. *Senior Nurse*, **3**, (1), 34–7.

Clawson, J.G. (1985) Is mentoring necessary? *Training Develop. J.*, **39**, (4), 36–9.

Clift, J.C. and Imrie, B.W. (1981) *Assessing Students and Appraising Teaching*, Croom Helm, London.

Clutterbuck, D. (1985) *Everybody Needs a Mentor: How To Further Talent Within an Organisation*, The Institute of Personnel Management, London.

Collins, N.W. (1983) *Professional Women and Their Mentors*, Prentice Hall, Englewood Cliffs, New Jersey.

Fagan, M.M. and Walter, G. (1982) Mentoring among teachers. *J. Educat. Res.*, **76**, (2), 113–18.

George, P. and Kummerow, J. (1981) Mentoring for career women. *Training*, **18**, (2), 44–9.

Hamilton, D. (1986) *Curriculum Evaluation*, 1976 Open Books, London.

Heron, J. (1973) *Experience and Method*, Human Potential Research Project, University of Surrey, Guildford, Surrey.

Holt, R. (1982) An alternative to mentorship. *Adult Education*, **55**, (2), 152–6.

Horney, K. (1962) *Self-Analysis*, Routledge and Kegan Paul, London.

Kanter, R.M. (1979) *Men and Women of the Corporation*, Basic Books, New York.

Klopf, G.J. and Harrison, J. (1981) Moving up the career ladder: the case for mentors. *Principal*, **61**, (1), 41–3.

McGregor, D. (1960) *The Human Side of Enterprise*, McGraw Hill, New York.

Merriam, S. (1984) Mentors and proteges: a critical review of the literature. *Adult Education Quarterly*, **33**, (3), 161–73.

Patton, M.Q. (1982) *Practical Evaluation*, Sage, Beverly Hills, Cal.

Phillip-Jones, L. (1982) *Mentors and Proteges*, Arbour House, New York.

Phillip-Jones, L. (1983) Establishing a formalised mentoring programme. *Training Develop. J.* (Feb), 38–42.

Rawlings, M.E. and Rawlings, L. (1983) Mentoring and networking for helping professionals. *Personnel Guidance J.*, **62**, (2), 116–18.

Roche, G.R. (1979) Much ado about mentors. *Harvard Business Review*, **56**, 14–28.

Rogers, J.C. (1982) Sponsorship – developing leaders for occupational therapy. *Amer. J. Occupat. Therapy*, **36**, 309–13.

Schmidt, J.A. and Wolfe, J.S. (1980) The mentor partnership: discovery of professionalism. *NASPA Journal*, **17**, 45–51.

Shamian, J. and Inhaber, R. (1985) The concept and practice of preceptorship in contemporary nursing: a review of pertinent literature. *The Intern. J. Nursing Studies*, **22**, (2), 79–88.

Shapiro, E.C., Haseltime, F. and Rowe, M. (1978) Moving up: role models, mentors and the patron system. *Sloan Management Review*, **19**, 51–8.

Simon, S.B., Howe, L.W. and Kirschenbaum, H. (1978) *Values Clarification: Revised Edition*, A and W visual Library, New York.

Speizer, J.J. (1981) Role models, mentors and sponsors: the elusive concept. *Signs*, **6**, 692–712.

Talyor, S. (1986) Mentors: who are they and what are they doing? *Thrust For Educational Leadership*, **15**, (7), 39–41.

CHAPTER FIVE: EDUCATIONAL PRINCIPLES AND CURRICULUM DESIGN IN EXPERIENTIAL LEARNING

Allan, D.M.E., Grosswald, S.J. and Means, R.P. (1984) Facilitating self-directed learning. In *Continuing Education for the Health Professions: Developing, Managing and Evaluating Programs for Maximum Impact on Patient Care* (eds J.S. Green S.J. Grosswald, E. Suter and D.B. Walthall), Jossey Bass, San Francisco, Cal.

Argyris, C. (1982) *Reasoning, Learning and Action*, Jossey Bass, San Francisco, Cal.

Argyris, C. and Schon, D. (1974) *Theory in Practice: Increasing Professional Effectiveness*, Jossey Bass, San Francisco, Cal.

Austin, E.K. (1981) *Guidelines for the Development of Continuing Education Offerings for Nurses*, Appleton-Century-Crofts, Norwalk, Conn.

Belbin, E. and Belbin, R.M. (1972) *Problems in Adult Retraining*, Heinemann, London.

Boud, D.J. (ed.) (1981) *Developing Student Autonomy in Learning*, Kogan Page, London.

Botkin, J., Elmandjra, M. and Malitza, M. (1979) *No Limits to Learning: Bridging the Human Gap*, Pergamon, London.

Brundage, D.H. and Mackeracher, D. (1980) *Adult Learning Principles and Their Application to Program Planning*, Ministry of Education, Ontario.

Bruner, J.S. (1966) *Towards a Theory of Instruction*, Bleknap, Cambridge, Mass.

Clark, M. (1978) Meeting the needs of the adult learner: using non-formal education for social action. *Convergence*, **XI**, 3–4.

Cross, K.P. (1981) *Adults as Learners*, Jossey Bass, San Francisco, Cal.

Cross-Durrant, A. (1984) Lifelong education in the writings of John Dewey. *Intern. J. Lifelong Education*, **3**, (2), 115–25.

Darkenwald, G.G. and Merriam, S.B. (1982) *Adult Education: Foundations of Practice*, Harper and Row, New York.

Elias, J.L. (1979) Andragogy revisited. *Adult Education*, **29**, 252–6.

Elias, J.L. and Merriam, S. (1980) *Philosophical Foundations of Adult Education*, Krieger, Flo.

Gordon, D. (1982) The Concept of the Hidden Curriculum. *Philosophy of Education*, **16**, (2), 187–8.

Houle, C.O. (1972) *The Design of Learning*, Jossey Bass, San Francisco, Cal.

Houle, C.O. (1984) *Patterns of Learning*, Jossey Bass, San Francisco, Cal.

Jarvis, P. (1983) *The Theory and Practice of Adult and Continuing Education*, Croom Helm, London.

Jarvis, P. (1985) *The Sociology of Adult and continuing Education*, Croom Helm, London.

Jenkins, D. and Shipman, M.D. (1976) *Curriculum: an Introduction*, Open Books, London.

Kidd, J.R. (ed.) (1973) *How Adults Learn*, Association Press, Chicago.

Knox, A.B. (1977) *Adult Development and Learning: a Handbook on Individual Growth and Competance in the Adult Years*, Jossey Bass, San Francisco, Cal.

Knox, A.B. (ed.) (1980) *Teaching Adults Effectively*, Jossey Bass, San Francisco, Cal.

Legge, D. (1982) *The Education of Adults in Britain*, Open University Press, Milton Keynes.

McCamiele, R. (ed.) (1982) *Calling Education Into Account*, Heinemann, London.

McIntosh, A. (1982) Psychology and Adult Education. In *Psychology in Practice* (eds S. Canter and D. Canter), Wiley, Chichester.

Mezeiro, J. (1981) A critical theory of adult learning and education. *Adult Education*, **32**, (1), 3–24.

Nadler, L. (ed.) (1984) *The Handbook of Human Resource Development*, Wiley, New York.

Niebuhr, H. (1977) *Revitalizing American Education: a New Approach that Might Just Work*, Wadsworth, Belmont, Cal.

Rogers, J. (ed.) (1977) *Adults Learning*, Open University Press, Milton Keynes.

Rogers, J. and Groombridge, B. (1976) *Right to Learn: The Case for Adult Equality*, Arrow, London.

Schon, D.A. (1983) *The Reflective Practioner: How Professionals Think in Action*, Basic Books, New York.

Index